From Syllable
to Conversation

FROM SYLLABLE TO CONVERSATION

Harris Winitz, Ph.D.
Professor of Speech Science and Psychology
University of Missouri-Kansas City

University Park Press
Baltimore • London • Tokyo

UNIVERSITY PARK PRESS
International Publishers in Science and Medicine
Chamber of Commerce Building
Baltimore, Maryland 21202

Copyright © 1975 by University Park Press

Typeset by The Composing Room of Michigan, Inc.
Printed in the United States of America by Universal Lithographers, Inc.
Second printing, September 1976

Library of Congress Cataloging in Publication Data

Winitz, Harris, 1933-
    From syllable to conversation.

    Bibliography: p.
    Includes index.
    1. Speech therapy. 2. Articulation disorders.
I. Title.
RC427.W56   616.8'55'06   75-29156
ISBN 0-8391-0893-2
ISBN 0-8391-0821-4 pbk.

Contents

Acknowledgment

I am deeply appreciative to my colleagues Conrad LaRiviere, Kay Mount, Stuart Ritterman, Marsha Zlatin, Elisabeth Wiig, Ralph Shelton, and James Reeds for their careful reading of the first draft. Although their helpful comments and suggestions are reflected in the text, the viewpoints and opinions are that of the author.

Preface

More than twenty years have passed since Robert Milisen and his associates (1954) completed the first serious study on articulatory behavior. At first the discipline was slow to respond, but in the early 1960's the pace began to quicken. As we look back it is difficult to imagine how research in the behavioral management of articulatory disorders could have been avoided, since our primary responsibility is to affect articulatory change.

Almost all of our constructs needed to be tested. Yet we failed to adopt the tools of the learning theorist. For example, we talked about the importance of discrimination training, but we never examined it. Strategies to reduce forgetting were never proposed. Acquisition and generalization were never tested.

This book is only a beginning, because we are only beginning to accumulate the facts. Nevertheless, it is time to assess what we know and how we can apply it.

From Syllable to Conversation examines each of the critical stages in articulatory training. First, the known facts are presented. Second, clinical applications are suggested. Third, clinical principles are given. At times I will move beyond the known, hoping that someday my proposals will be subject to empirical test.

This book is written for both students and professionals; students will have the opportunity to learn the origin of clinical routines, and professionals will have the challenge of matching their suppositions against mine. From all of this can only come progress and eventually a sturdy science on which the clinical management of articulatory disorders can rest.

Harris Winitz
Professor, Speech Science and Psychology

for Flora Sue, Simeon, and Jennifer, and
all His children who use language as if
they made it

CHAPTER 1

Searching for a Perspective

If there were no published works on the treatment of articulatory disorders, what operational procedures would one devise? Essentially this question was raised by the early writers of our profession. It was apparent to them that three major dimensions should be explored: a) evaluation of the disorder, b) background or cause of the disorder, and c) establishment of treatment procedures to reduce or eliminate the disorder. Each one of these areas of study does not lead to obvious solutions.

EVALUATION

Evaluation usually begins with description. We might, then, ask the question: How should we describe articulatory errors? This question is important because the descriptions we use will affect the way we evaluate and treat articulation disorders. One obvious system is simply to list the sounds in error and the error types.

Let us assume a child manifests the following articulation errors:

Correct sound	Error sound
/θ/	/t/
/ð/	/d/
/s/	/t/
/z/	/d/
/f/	/p/
/v/	/b/

We could simply stop at this point and ask no further questions. What basis would we have for treatment? We would know which sounds are in error as well as the errors of substitution, but how would we proceed from here? A list of the error sounds does not tell us how to develop a training program; it only tells us which sounds are in error.

Early writers (Van Riper, 1939; Ainsworth, 1948) additionally recommended that error types should be catalogued. Usually, error types were partitioned as follows:

1. *Substitution:* one sound replaces another sound (/t/ for /k/)
2. *Distortion:* the target sound is altered slightly and is usually not regarded as a standard English sound (a lateral lisp for /s/)
3. *Omission:* the target sound is absent (pronouncing spill as /pɪl/)

At least two questions immediately emerge: What is the operational difference between substitution and distortion, and what value is this classification system?

Substitution versus Distortion

With regard to the first question, substitution and distortion, it can be said that the term distortion is usually employed to denote a substitution which is an uncommon English sound. Van Riper (1972, p. 187) takes this position when he says that "distortions are substitutions of sounds foreign to our language . . . ."

A lateral lisp is often referred to as a distortion of /s/. Distortions can be described rather easily with phonetic symbols. A lateralized substitution is an /l/ which is voiceless, like the /l/ in the word slow, but made with considerably more frication. The standard phonetic symbol for the voiceless lateral fricative is [ɬ]. The little open circle below the /l/ indicates that the sound is voiceless.

The use of the term distortion implies more than a definition. It really involves an evaluation, and, therefore, points of disagreement are sure to surface regarding what is an approximation (a slight distortion) of an English sound.

Let us assume that a young child aspirates /k/ when it follows /s/. At this point we will define aspiration as a small puff of air following the release of /k/. Usually /k/ is aspirated in the initial word position and in several other environments, but never after /s/. Thus the pronunciation of [skʰeɪt] for "skate" would be regarded as incorrect. Note that the ʰ after /k/ means that /k/ is aspirated. Try saying it this way. Pronounce the /h/ in [kʰeɪt] with considerable aspiration, and at the same time place your hand in front of your mouth and you will feel a slight breath of air. The air cannot be felt when the word skate is uttered in its usual way.

Young children often aspirate /k/ after /s/ as they are learning English. Should we regard the k^h/k pronunciation as a substitution or a distortion? Does it really matter? It may depend upon what conclusions we wish to draw. This brings us to the second issue raised above, that is, the value of the classification system.

Classification

To my knowledge the categories of substitution, distortion, and omission are non-functional, in that their predictive value has never been tested. As of now, improvement cannot be prejudged on the basis of error type.

It would be relatively easy to examine the practical utility of these three error types if children could be found to fit these categories. Let us assume that we are able to find children who evidenced only one of the three error types for the /s/ sound. The following groups might be selected for investigation:

Group I: omission of /s/
Group II: lateral distortion of /s/
Group III: /θ/ substitution of /s/

Children in each of the three groups would then participate in a training program in which they would be taught to produce the /s/ sound correctly. From this experiment we would realize information regarding the relation between error type and the learning of /s/, the target sound.

Returning now to the example of the child's articulation errors given at the start of the chapter, we might consider descriptions other than error type. We might pay attention to the fact that the target sounds are all fricatives and the errors are all stops (plosives). It would seem, then, that only one phonetic feature is consistently being misused. Perhaps consistency of misarticulation is something to consider when we plan our program of instruction.

Other considerations that may influence the selection of treatment procedures relate to levels of performance. Can the child imitate one or more of the target sounds? Does his error type reflect a consistent substitution? Does he misarticulate only in sentences, but not in single words?

Evaluation as Data Gathering

The evaluation can be regarded as a data-gathering experiment. The information one seeks should be guided by the research findings of carefully executed investigations. When there is no information clearly pertinent to the child or adult whom you are treating, you may wish to make observations in areas of your own personal experience. However, you would not want to make observations or administer tests in order to obtain information that clearly is not relevant or significant according to all of the available literature sources. Without research investigations, our evaluations would be intuitive and without principled direction.

BACKGROUND

In addition to studying the client's articulatory performance, speech clinicians often recommend that background information be made available to the clinician. A host of considerations at first seem important. These might include: a) health and personality of the client and his family, b) intelligence of the client, c) hearing and motor coordination of the client, and d) the social and educational background of the client.

This text is concerned with the mechanics of articulatory production for children who do not evidence an organic pathology. For this reason we will only briefly consider background or etiological considerations. Factors that should be included in an initial evaluation have been summarized previously (Winitz, 1969). In some instances the attitudes of parents should be assessed, as the research of Sommers and his colleagues (Sommers et al., 1964) suggests. When these attitudes are determined to be detrimental to a child's success, parental counseling is recommended. The social and psychological environments are important considerations when treating children with articulation disorders. The fact that this dimension is not covered in this text should not imply that it is unimportant.

Determining the cause of an articulation error, when an organic pathology is not present, is extremely difficult and in the past has largely proved to be non-productive. Discussions of causes are frequent (Van Riper, 1939, 1972; Winitz, 1969; Powers, 1971). In general, however, the available research does not point securely and easily to underlying etiologies of articulation disorders.

Articulatory Errors Resulting from Approximations

After an exhaustive search of many studies in this area (Winitz, 1969), I offered the tentative conclusion that articulation errors represent learned behavior. Several years ago I took the point of view that approximations become stabilized in the speech of young children. Children usually do not pronounce words correctly when they are learning to talk. Some sounds are misarticulated, and syllables are often deleted.

There may be several reasons why children utter word approximations. One reason, which is treated in greater detail later, may be that words are used before phonetic mastery is complete. Having heard a word a relatively few times, a child may not be able to internalize all of the phonetic and phonological rules that govern it. Another possibility is that sounds must be practiced before they are perfected. If practice is essential, it seems reasonable to expect that the early utterances will be slightly off "target." With more practice, the target sounds will be acquired.

It is generally recognized that the early words of children (Lewis, 1951; Albright and Albright, 1958; Winitz and Irwin, 1958; Smith, 1973) are only approximations of the standard word. Listed below are word approximations observed by Smith (1973) in the speech of his two-year-old child:

Approximation	Standard word
[dɛp]	stamp
[dɛt]	tent
[gɛu:]	thank you
[b̥igik]	biscuit
[ʌgu]	uncle
[b̥i:]	please
[nu:]	nose

The small open circle signifies devoicing of a stop normally voiced. Unlike the voiceless stops, these sounds are unaspirated and lax.

Approximations sometimes can end up as articulatory errors. Smith (1973) observed the occurrence of the lateral lisp in his son's speech as a substitution for the /sl/ blend at about two years, nine months. Up to this point the /s/ was omitted and /sl/ initial words began only with /l/ (e.g., [lʌg] for "slug"). The child's attempt to pronounce /sl/ correctly apparently led to the adding of frication and devoicing of /l/, resulting in [ɬ], the lateral lisp. This voiceless lateral fricative generalized almost immediately to all /sl-/contexts, but not to other /s/-consonant contexts, such as /st/ and /sm/. Shortly thereafter, the lateral lisp generalized to a few words beginning with /s/. As an example, we can trace the chronology of pronunciations for the word silver:

Pronunciation	Age
[wɪvə]	2 years, 5 months
[lɪvlə]	2 years, 7 months
[ɬɪvlə]	2 years, 9 months
[sɪvlə]	3 years, 1.5 months
[silvə]	3 years, 4.5 months

Almost immediately after [ɬ] appeared for /sl/ at two years, nine months, it replaced the initial /l/ in the word silver. The lateral fricative was retained for almost four and one-half months, or until three years, one and one-half months.

It is of interest to note that Smith's child pronounced /sn-/ clusters with an initial [n̥]. The [n̥], like the [ɬ], is a frequent substitution for /s/. In addition, Smith's son had a great number of substitutions for the /r/. Frequently observed were [w], [l], and [d]. All of these sounds are common substitutions for the /r/ sound.

Although there is no strong evidence indicating that articulatory errors emerge from approximations, there seems to be no way to dispute it at this time. If the findings obtained by Smith (1973) can be generalized, they suggest that the etiological foundation of articulatory errors can be easily traced to early sound substitutions. Why some children retain these errors, while others do not, is difficult to explain, although we have speculated that the explanation resides in the parent-child interaction and cannot be accounted for by etiologies housed within the child's brain and vocal tract.

Like Smith's child, other children have been observed to have sound productions that are variable. At times the target sound is correct, and at other times it is incorrect. The same is true of children with articulatory errors. In some phonetic contexts, they produce the sound incorrectly, and in others they produce the sound correctly. Sometimes, however, a few children consistently misarticulate a sound. In Chapter 2, we summarize the findings of an investigation by McReynolds and Huston (1971) demonstrating that, for sounds consistently in error, the phonetic features that make up the sound are usually uttered correctly when other sounds are considered. But more about this interesting study later.

There is general consensus that articulation errors are variable. However, there is no interpretation regarding the maintenance of errors that is affirmatively agreed upon by all. My interpretation is that inconsistency can be traced to early word approximations that have persisted. Perhaps the most obvious reason for the maintenance of errors can be found in the relationship between parent and child. A parent who listens without rephrasing error-filled sentences gives his child only half a chance. A parent who acknowledges understanding mispronounced words rewards incorrect pronunciations. Conceivably, then, the more tolerant the parent is of deviant speech, the more likely is the chance that his child will make no attempt to alter pronunciations.

I know scholars who pronounced the word et cetera as /ɛksɛtərə/ and did not alter this pronunciation until they were told it was incorrect.

External monitoring seems important especially when pronunciation becomes fixed after several years of use.

Value of Background Information

Let us now turn to the problem we hinted to above, the practical utility of the background information for children who evidence no organic pathology as determined by a physician. Assuming the information we have collected is accurate, we are faced with the responsibility to use it. If a child, for example, scores poorly on a motor test of rhythm or a test of social skills, we are obligated to do something about it, or we should not have sought the information in the first place. We might recommend certain motor exercises or prescribe a series of social readiness sessions. In practice, clinicians often disregard their own test taking. This routine is a curious fact, but it is fairly general across clinicians.

Often children with a number of articulation errors, seem normal in examinations given by psychologists and physicians. Even so, some diagnosticians frequently make one of the following two conclusions: a) the child seems normal in all respects except for his speech, or b) the child seems normal, but there are indications of minimal impairments. To be sure, these reports differ in interpretation, not in fact. In some settings, it is becoming fashionable to recommend that there are "soft neurological signs" rather than to admit that the expensive examinations have led only to a larger medical bill.

When our colleagues from other health professions recommend "minimal impairment" as a diagnosis, it is tempting to begin a series of in-house motor and social tests (see Winitz, 1969, Powers, 1971). If a child performs below average, it is also tempting to conclude that his score suggests an impairment or disability. Once we conclude that there is an impairment, we are obligated to treat it before training is initiated. If not, why conduct the tests?

Although many clinicians will not easily give up their determination to find a cause, they seem not to take their investigations seriously. Most of the time, they will go ahead and begin to modify the speech errors without regard to the findings of their evaluation, unless it is clear that a serious physical abnormality (cleft palate, cerebral palsy, etc.) or emotional disturbance (autism) exists.

Past investigations have demonstrated that, with the exception of measures of speech sound discrimination, articulatory defective children and normal speaking children perform equally well on tests of physical and emotional maturity (Winitz, 1969). This point was highlighted in the introduction of a recent paper by Yoss and Darley (1974, p. 399), stating, ". . . the etiology of functional articulation disorders remains undetermined." We are in agreement with their position, yet it is a curious fact that this investigation by Yoss and Darley is prototypical of those that generate inconclusive statements. My only reason for singling out this paper is because it is recent and well done, except for an error in the selection of subjects. Poor control in the selection of subjects makes a good study turn sour.

Selection of Subjects

The Yoss and Darley investigation, like so many in the past, compares normal speaking and articulatory defective speaking children on a variety of speech and facial tasks. Among the tests included by the authors, three are listed below:

1. Isolated volitional oral movements: blowing, puffing of cheeks, whistling, and others
2. Sequenced volitional oral movements: imitation of sequences of oral movements, such as puckering the lips and wagging the tongue from side to side
3. Diadochokinetic rate: repetition of syllables and syllable sequences—/pʌ/, /tʌ/, /kʌ/, and /pʌ tə kə/

When differences are obtained between normal and defective speaking children on tasks similar to those used by Yoss and Darley, a number of interpretations can be offered. One simple interpretation is that there are maturational differences between the groups. Essentially this conclusion was drawn by Yoss and Darley (p. 412). They state, "The findings . . . lend substantial support to the use of the term 'developmental apraxia of speech' as descriptive of their articulatory problem." Apraxia can be defined as a loss in the ability to program the speech musculature for volitional productions of speech sounds. As we will soon see, the conclusion drawn by Yoss and Darley is untenable.

Another interpretation which can be made is that the neurologies of the two speaking groups are different. Yoss and Darley avoided this problem by saying (p. 411), " 'Soft' neurologic findings of uncertain significance or equivocal clinical importance do not imply a pathologic condition of the central nervous system, nor can one say that such findings imply minimal brain damage or minimal cerebral dysfunction." What do "soft" signs imply? To Yoss and Darley, they imply a developmental lag, which apparently is not reflective of the integrity of the central nervous system.

Fortunately, we do not need to untie the knots that Yoss and Darley have woven, for their investigation suggests a second interpretation: The experimental subjects are basically different from the control subjects. We do not know the origin of the experimental subjects, only that they were screened at the well known Mayo Clinic. We are told that the subjects' articulatory productions "constituted a clinical, social, or academic problem or warranted enrollment in speech therapy" (p. 401).

The control subjects were carefully selected so as to resemble the experimental subjects, but it is not clear what procedures were used to select them. If they were taken from community schools, comparisons with defective speaking children would be unfair. The defective speaking children may have been brought to the Mayo Clinic for reasons in addition to their speech errors. They may have been representative of a population of children with learning disabilities. Perhaps the children had social and psychological problems.

Sketched below is the selection procedure for the ideal control and experimental group if the Yoss and Darley investigation were to be replicated:

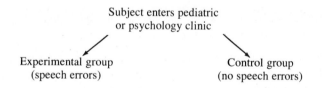

Subject enters pediatric
or psychology clinic

Experimental group   Control group
(speech errors)   (no speech errors)

If these procedures were routinely followed as subjects were assigned to the control and experimental groups, then differences that emerged could be attributed to basic differences in the subject population. At the present time, it is difficult to conclude that the experimental subjects evidenced retardation in isolated and sequenced volitional movements, inasmuch as it is possible that their low scores may have reflected social, psychological, and developmental dysfunctions.

TREATMENT

As indicated above, our discussion of treatment is restricted to the mechanics of articulatory modification. Procedures of modification are really speech tools that speech clinicians use to bring about change in the articulation of their clients. It is of interest that not everyone looks at this process in the same way.

Importance of Controlled Experimentation

Moskowitz (1972) commented rather directly against procedures that I recommended (Winitz, 1969) because to her they reflect artificialities and superficities. The position that Moskowitz holds is stated as follows (Moskowitz, 1972, p. 495):

> Many of the techniques discussed here [in Winitz, 1969] have probably been very useful in producing the kind of learning that speech therapists [sic] have attempted to attain for handicapped children: but what, in fact, are they teaching? It seems to me that where they are successful, they are only superficially so, as no technique seriously considers the need of the individual child.

Further on, Moskowitz dismisses controlled research studies by citing a personal experience with a clinical population. She reviewed the work of a teacher of the deaf with the following comments (Moskowitz, 1972, p. 496):

> Using a variety of techniques which might be considered outlandish by some, usually designed on the spot to fit the exact needs of a particular student, Zemalis has managed to teach students with congenital deafness to pronounce English well enough to communicate and practice their trades . . .

And still later, Moskowitz (1972, p. 497) summarizes her reaction to controlled experimentation on treatment by remarking:

> The closer we can come to facilitating the child's normal abilities, rather than substituting artificial speedy techniques, the more useful will be our teaching.

Thus, it seems that Moskowitz prefers "outlandish techniques designed on the spot" to experiments that carefully select and study treatment variables. At no point does Moskowitz define the terms "normal" or "artificial," and her failure to do so means that she wishes to ignore data. Her biases cannot be entertained seriously, for she fails to define terms, ignores research findings, and fails to act constructively.

Moskowitz reflects a position shared by many when behavioral technology was introduced to the field of speech pathology over ten years ago. People argued about what was *natural*. Instead, they should have asked: What established principles of learning theory and of normal language development should be considered in the preparation of clinical techniques? The major goal of behavioral technology, as it applies to speech pathology, is to functionalize the teaching environment for children who have experienced failure. How do we know what will produce an optimal learning experience? One obvious way is to conduct laboratory experiments.

Laboratory experiments are conducted to squeeze out relevant variables, and machines are often used to deliver and count stimuli in order to increase precision. When variables are found to be significant under controlled conditions, we can presume they will continue to be effective under conditions that are less than ideal. That their prepotency will be slightly diminished when conditions are less than perfect is, of course, acknowledged. Nevertheless, we cannot discount the overriding importance of systematic exploration.

The clinical procedures presented in the following chapters are guiding principles to be implemented under a variety of educational environments. There is no suggestion that procedures employed in experiments should prescribe exactly clinical routines. A case in point is reinforcement. In order to gain precision, investigators may use token reinforcers rather than social reinforcers. In the setting of an experiment, a child may be given a penny or a piece of candy each time he responds correctly. However, we should not assume that the experimenter is advocating the use of candy in a clinical situation, only that correct articulatory productions should be recognized and acknowledged.

When one takes the position that experimental procedures serve as models of learning experiences that clinicians can provide, the reservations Moskowitz holds can be dismissed. However, we cannot dismiss experimentation; for without it, teaching techniques would have no principled basis.

Treatment Considerations

With this rather lengthy defense of the experimental approach, we shall now discuss treatment considerations. As discussed in the first section, before articulatory training is begun, the level of articulatory functioning needs to be assessed. We need to know at what point articulatory performance breaks down. For example, pronunciation may be excellent in isolated words, but articulatory errors may be frequent in conversation. Or a child may be able to pronounce a sound when asked to imitate, but not when he is asked to describe an object or read.

Although we will outline the various stages in the treatment process, we should remember that it is not essential to bring each child through the entire training sequence. The sequence presented below is simply a start-to-finish program. For individual children, only certain segments might need to be emphasized.

The learning of articulatory responses can be segmented into essentially four processes: a) discrimination training, b) production practice, c) transfer of training, and d) retention. In discrimination training, children are taught to distinguish between speech sounds or segments. After they can successfully distinguish between important phonetic elements, they are given practice in producing sounds or sound sequences. They are also taught to generalize their production skills to new contexts and environments. Finally, they are given practice in the recall of sounds in full sentences and in conversational situations.

It should be emphasized that the sequence of training is not fixed. It may be necessary, for example, to teach discrimination of sounds in sentences long after the sound is acquired in isolated words. In fact, it is possible that the failure to emphasize discrimination training at this level is a significant omission in our current clinical routines.

In this text, full attention is given to the behavioral processes of discrimination, production, transfer, and retention. In addition, consideration is given to articulation testing, distinctive features, and coarticulation because these concepts are importantly related to the four behavioral processes emphasized in the text. We begin our discussion by introducing the topic of distinctive features.

CHAPTER 2

Features and Their Role in Articulatory Training

Feature systems are beginning to have an important impact on the development of clinical programs (Compton 1970; Singh and Polen, 1972; McReynolds and Engmann, 1975; Singh, in press). For this reason a full chapter is devoted to this topic. In this chapter and in the following chapters, continuing use of phonetic features will be made, as we discuss treatment variables.

CONCEPT OF FEATURE

What is a feature? It is a relatively simple concept, although the specification of features is not always an easy task, and, in some instances, there is considerable disagreement among linguistic scientists. A feature can be thought of as a segment of a stimulus complex, and, as we will soon acknowledge, the segment can be used at an abstract level.

Consider, for example, the following stimulus complexes. Can you recognize one feature common to both of them?

The geometric forms have an X placed above them. Consider the following geometric forms. They both have the letter Y placed below them.

It is easy to distinguish between X and non-X pairs, and just as easy to describe them. We can refer to the circles in the following ways: the circle with the X, the circle without the X, the circle with the Y, and the circle without the Y. In all cases the presence or absence of the X or Y is the distinguishing feature.

Let us denote the presence of the X by [+X] and the absence of the X by [−X]. Using symbols such as these, the circles, as well as the squares, can be distinguished in the following ways:

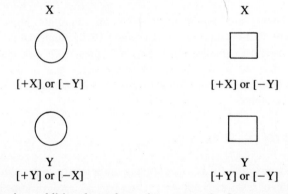

By employing additional markers the geometric forms can be further distinguished:

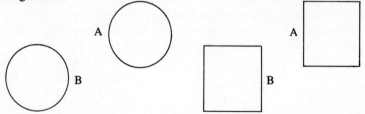

Using the letter markers A, B, X, and Y, circles, for example, can be distinguished in the following ways:

Geometric form   *Feature specification*

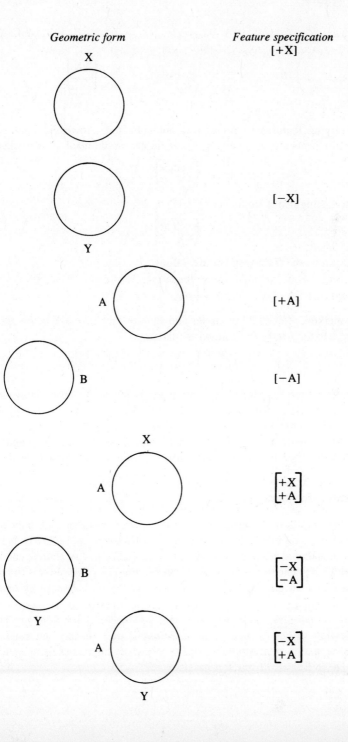

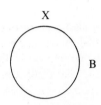

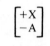

In specifying features [+circle] was not indicated. However, since two geometric forms are involved, X, for example, would need to be marked:

$$\begin{bmatrix} +\text{circle} \\ +\text{X} \end{bmatrix}$$

so as to distinguish it from:

$$\begin{bmatrix} -\text{circle} \\ +\text{X} \end{bmatrix}$$

Examine the following feature values:

$$\begin{bmatrix} -\text{X} \\ +\text{A} \end{bmatrix}$$

These markers refer to those circles and squares that have a Y below them and an A to their left. The following markers:

$$\begin{bmatrix} +\text{Y} \\ +\text{B} \end{bmatrix}$$

refer to those circles and squares that have the labels Y and B. However, [+Y] and [+B] can be specified by using the values [−X] and [−A], respectively, indicating that only the markers X and A need to be used. Modern linguistic theory defines each marker as having a + and − specification. This is because each marker is viewed as bipolar in form.

Application to Phonetics

There are similarities between the above letter markers and phonetic features. For example, we can refer to a nasal sound as [+nasal] and a non-nasal sound as [−nasal] (or [+oral] in English), just as a circle can be [+X] or [−X]. The symbol system of modern linguistics employs + and − specifications for each feature, rather than specifying a feature by using two + marks: [+X] and [+Y] for the example above, or [+nasal] and [+oral] for nasality, and [+voiced] and [+voiceless] for voicing. The specification values + and −, as in [+nasal] or [−nasal], are used to denote the quality or attribute of nasality, which distinguishes nasal sounds (/m, n, ŋ/ in English) from non-nasal sounds.

Let us assume, for example, that a young child has difficulty producing nasal sounds. After careful study the following rule is developed to describe errors of the nasal sounds: nasal sounds are deleted in final position before voiced stops. For this child, then, the word can is pronounced /kæ/ in "can go," and the word seem is pronounced /si/ in "seem different."

If nasals do not appear before voiced stops, how do we know that they have been deleted? It is because they appear in all other contexts, such as "can see" and "seem wide." Further justification for assuming that the abstract forms of "can" and "seem" end with a nasal comes from the observation that the vowels of these words are usually nasalized, although admittedly this observation would not necessarily be important for all phonologists.

The abstract form of the word can is /kæn/, but a common phonetic variation is [kæ̃]. We can summarize this situation as follows:

Underlying form, phonemic level	Phonetic level
/kæn/	[kæ̃]

Rule: *The sequence [+nasal] [+stop]—that is, a nasal followed by a stop—results in the deletion of the nasal consonant.*

Another example might be helpful here. It is clear to all speakers of American English that the intervocalic /t/ sound—/t/ occurring between two vowels—is not the same as /t/ produced in other phonetic contexts. In intervocalic position the /t/ changes to a number of phonetic forms, most often to an [r]-flap, a quick movement of the front of the tongue toward and away from the alveolar region. We can illustrate this point as follows:

Phonemic level	Phonetic level
/bɛtər/	[bɛřər]

Rule: */t/ becomes [ř] in intervocalic position.*

Let us give another example of an underlying form. Suppose a child substitutes /t/ for /s/ and /θ/, /d/ for /z/ and /ð/, /p/ for /f/, and /b/ for /v/. It is clear that the error sounds all have something in common: Front fricatives are substituted by stops.

Rule: $\begin{bmatrix} +fricative \\ +front \end{bmatrix}$ *becomes* [−fricative].

It is not difficult to see, then, that features are convenient tools for describing phonetic events at various levels of abstraction. Linguists use the term *distinctive features* when they describe the structure of abstract phonological entities, although the features they employ vary somewhat from those used in this text. We will continue to use those features familiar to you, while trying to do justice to new and exciting concepts.

Abstract Phonetic Level

The phonetic level can be regarded as a link between the abstract phonological level and the mechanisms that produce speech. Although abstract, the phonetic level contains considerably more detail than high order phonological levels. At the phonetic level, the binary trait often gives way to more concrete specifications. The feature nasality, as an illustration, might be specified as nasal, partially nasal, or non-nasal (Kent, Carney, and Severeid, 1974).

Recently, phonologists have reinterpreted the phonetic level. It is no longer regarded as simply an abstraction of the articulations of speech, but as the final phases of the phonological description of speech sequences.

Phoneticians have long recognized that phonetic transcription falls far short of a play-by-play description of the movement of the speech articulators. This point was cogently conveyed by Chao (1968, p. 46) when he told the following story:

> ...a Swiss lecturer who spoke no English once came to New York and delivered a lecture from notes written in IPA [the International Phonetic Alphabet] and the audience could not understand a word he said.

Speech pathologists, as they go about preparing treatment procedures, sometimes assume that the phonetic level is a description of productions. Perhaps for this reason speech gestures are often viewed as static rather than dynamic in form. In this text, both static (features) and dynamic (movements) considerations are taken into account. Emphasis is on the gestural components of neighboring sounds that, in some cases, should be considered as individual sounds are taught. This is discussed in detail in Chapter 6.

DISTINCTIVE FEATURE THEORY

At this point it is important to reconsider the term distinctive feature. Distinctive features are those phonetic elements (see Jakobson, Fant, and Halle, 1952; Chomsky and Halle, 1968) that have been found to be appropriate for describing the phonological rules of the many natural languages of the world. In addition, distinctive features are binary in form; that is, each feature has a + and a − specification.

Phonological Universals

Let us pause for a moment to examine these two qualities. An aim of linguistic theory is the discovery of universal laws of grammar. A universal law is one that is language independent: It applies to all languages. The discovery of a universal rule in linguistics is as exciting as finding a "constant" in the physical sciences. The foundation of all sciences, linguistics included, rests on the discovery of basic laws.

We indicated in our definition of distinctive features that the term distinctive applies to those features that have been found to be "appropriate for describing phonological rules." Changes are to be expected and, of course, continue to be recommended (Ladefoged, 1971). Scientific theories often seem as neat as the parallel printed lines and justified margins in which they appear. Distinctive feature theory is no exception. We can anticipate revision in the features and, perhaps, in some of the underlying constructs.

Bipolar Features

The binary structure of distinctive features has been found to be convenient for the description of phonological rules. A feature, then, has two heads, or if you prefer, a head and a tail. Let us pursue this point further with the nasality feature.

As indicated above, the nasality feature has the bipolar specifications [+nasal] and [−nasal]. We can now introduce a rule involving nasal consonants. The following rule is simply for illustrative purposes, although it is probably applicable to a large number of languages. The rule, which applies to consonants, is as follows:

Rule: *For consonants, [+nasal] becomes [−voice] following [−voice].*

A great number of sequences are governed by this rule, some of which are listed below:

/sn/ becomes [sn̥]
/tn/ becomes [tn̥]
/kn/ becomes [kn̥]
/fn/ becomes [fn̥]
/θm̥/ becomes [θm̥]
/ʃɹ/ becomes [ʃɹ̥]

Not all of these sound sequences occur in every language, but for those languages having the sequence [−voice] [+nasal], this rule would probably apply.

In classical phonetic theory, the presence of a feature value generally implies the absence of a contrastive value. A sound which is nasal cannot be oral, and a sound which is bilabial cannot be labiodental. In the feature system developed by Jakobson, Fant, and Halle (1952) and refined by Chomsky and Halle (1968), the dichotomous values ([+nasal] and [+voice], etc.) are explicitly stated. Each feature is viewed as binary, having a + value and a − value. In contrast to other more phonetically based feature systems, the binary poles are explicit. For example, in the Jakobson, Fant, and Halle system, the grave-acute feature distinguishes labials from dentals:

Grave consonants	Acute consonants
m	n
f	s
p	θ
v	t
b	z
	ð
	d

Although velars were regarded as grave, and palatals as acute, in the original formulations of Jakobson, Fant, and Halle, they remained unspecified with regard to English segments until a later reformulation by Halle (1964a):

Grave consonants	Acute consonants
p	t
b	d
m	θ
f	ð
v	n
k	s
g	z
	tʃ
	dʒ
	ʃ
	ʒ

Grave, as we can see above, refers to sounds articulated in the periphery of the oral cavity (labials and velars), whereas *acute* refers to an articulation closure or narrowing in the medial region of the oral cavity (palatals-dentals-alveolars). In spelling out the oppositions, in what seems to be a cohesive and unified way, the negative values are assigned to a particular set of sounds. In classical phonetic systems the − value, or negative value, is unspecified. It generally refers to all sounds with the exception of the + value, or positively stated segments. However, for feature systems that reflect the influence of Jakobson, all sounds are specified on the + and − range.

It also should be pointed out that Jakobsonian systems are not phonetic systems, but arrangements designed to capture the abstractions of phonetic events across languages. The phonetic level is not ignored in these systems. Rather, in many instances the phonetic events, from which the phonological abstractions are made, are clearly indicated. The phonetic level of these systems often includes additional phonetic detail as well as new features that have not appeared as elements in the abstract phonological levels. For example, in English, aspiration would remain unspecified until the phonetic level. It is a distinctive feature, since it is distinctive in languages other than English, but the aspiration feature does not need to be specified in English in order to formulate abstract phonological rules.

Again, it is important to stress that, although the phonetic level is more descriptive than the phonological level which dominates it, the phonetic level is not a model of speech production. A description of the several levels of articulatory encoding is given in Chapter 6, where the differences between the phonological and phonetic levels are again emphasized.

History

Admittedly, interest in distinctive feature theory as a useful methodology for serious study of articulation disorders is recent, but such need not have been the case. It is difficult to deny that distinctive feature theory—whether of the genre of Jakobson, Fant, and Halle (1952) and Chomsky and Halle (1968), or of other investigators—has had a profound impact on the way clinical questions are now being framed. Yet many of the current investigations could have been conducted long before the term "distinctive feature" became fashionable in clinical circles. In particular, investigations involving behavioral manipulation of phonetic segments could have been handled within the traditional phonetic classifications of voicing, and place and manner of articulation. Admittedly, these studies might evidence weaknesses by contemporary linguistic standards. Yet the recognition that, in many instances, articulatory errors were non-random, led early investigators to recommend the use of rules for describing the phonetic behavior of children (Albright and Albright, 1958; House, 1961).

If feature theory could have been applied many years ago, why has it only recently been used? The reason cannot be determined with certainty, although there seems to be an explanation. Increased interest in the theory of behavioral modification led to the question of what to modify. It became increasingly clear that features and the way in which they are organized should be carefully considered in clinical programs.

In all fairness, it should be mentioned that recognition of production segments (or features) has not been ignored in the clinical practice of articulation. Van Riper's (1939) suggestion to teach the movements of "thrusting," "blowing," "curling," or "grooving," as preparatory exercises when teaching sounds, was clear recognition in the early years of our profession that sounds are composed of segments or features of production. However, the clinical methodologies that evolved from such suggestions were sterile, consisting only of lists of prescriptive routines having no foundation in physiological or psychological phonetics.

PROBLEMS IN THE USE OF FEATURE SYSTEMS

It is now important to consider a number of issues raised by Walsh (1974) in his recently published article. Walsh makes a number of significant points, which should be carefully evaluated since interest in feature systems is high.

First, Walsh took issue with the use of the term feature as I (Winitz, 1969) and others wrote about it. At certain points I used the term feature when referring to both the + and − values of the Jakobsonian features. I was mostly concerned with introducing this new system, and, in one or two places, use of the term feature for one of the bipolar attributes was intentional, although I see now that it has been a source of confusion. Walsh is clearly correct in saying that when one refers to binary features, as they have been developed by Jakobson, Fant, and Halle (1952) and Chomsky and Halle (1968), the + and − specifications cannot be called features.

We can illustrate this point by listing as an example the nasality and voicing features and their specifications:

Feature	Specifications
Nasality	[+nasal], [−nasal]
Voicing	[+voice], [−voice]

The term feature has been used in several ways, as Liberman et al. (1967) have remarked. For the most part, throughout this text the term refers to production segments, such as nasal and non-nasal, voiced and voiceless. In the context in which we are employing these terms, we anticipate no misinterpretation. The term feature as used in this text, then, can be thought of as a target value of articulatory events—the manner, place, and voicing segments of speech sounds.

Second, Walsh contends that distinctive features do not provide precise enough phonetic based data to be useful in clinical research. To make this point clear, let us refer to an important article by McReynolds and Huston (1971), where children with severe articulatory deviations were examined. Many of the sounds were consistently incorrect; that is, they were never produced correctly even though they were tested in a great number of phonetic and word environments.

Let us examine one child about whom McReynolds and Huston reported in detail, and who was representative of the children in their study. After intensive examination, some sounds were never found to be produced correctly. Some of these sounds were: /t, d, f, v, θ, s, z, ʃ, ʒ/.

Next, McReynolds and Huston examined the sounds that were produced correctly and made special note of their features. McReynolds and Huston made use of the Chomsky and Halle (1968) system, and it is for this reason that they drew the fire of Walsh (1974).

The finding of the McReynolds and Huston (1971) investigation showed that stridency was the single feature misused by this child. All other features (really their articulatory correlates) appeared at one time or another as a segment of a correctly produced sound. For example, although tongue tip to alveolar movement might be missing in /t, d, s/, it appeared in other phonetic units, such as in the correctly articulated /n/ sound. McReynolds and Huston concluded that features not produced in target sounds will appear in the productions of other sounds.

The approach taken by McReynolds and Huston raises at least two issues that need to be explored: a) the appropriateness of the feature system, and b) the implication of these findings for clinical instruction.

Appropriateness of Feature System

With regard to the first issue, Walsh maintains that the features of the Chomsky-Halle system are too abstract to provide meaningful data to validate the consideration rasied by McReynolds and Huston. The features are abstract, precisely because they have been designed to elucidate abstract relationships, both ''phonetic'' and grammatical, both within and across languages. Features can be converted into phonetic segments, but as they are defined and used in phonology they are not phonetic units in the usual sense.

Important phonetic facts are, of course, recoverable when the Chomsky-Halle system is applied to English. For example, consider the several ways in which a /θ/ for /s/ substitution can be described:

Sound change
/s/ becomes /θ/

Feature change[1] (Chomsky-Halle)   *Feature change (Traditional-phonetic)*

$$\begin{bmatrix} + \text{strident} \\ - \text{high} \\ + \text{coronal} \\ - \text{voice} \end{bmatrix}$$

becomes [−strident]

$$\begin{bmatrix} + \text{alveolar} \\ + \text{fricative} \\ - \text{voice} \end{bmatrix}$$

becomes [+dental]

In both feature systems the phonetic facts reflecting the θ/s substitution are clear, but the Chomsky-Halle system is more abstract in that the phonetic specifications of stridency would need to be defined. We recall that the major finding of McReynolds and Huston was: Features not available in target sounds can be found in other productions. For this finding to have clinical utility, Walsh contends, the feature needs to be concrete—as close as possible to a physiological gesture.

In most instances, the Chomsky-Halle features cause no difficulty in making interpretations about production, but there are occasions, as Walsh suggests, that are unresolvable.

This point can be illustrated well with the stridency and anterior features. Consider the stridency feature first. According to the (phonetic) interpretation given by McReynolds and Huston, the "percentage of correct usage" of [+strident], for the child reported above, would be zero. The "percentage of correct usage" for [−strident] would be greater than zero, since [−strident] applies not only to the two fricatives /θ/ and /ð/, but to stops, nasals, and semivowels as well.

Classifying the fricatives as [−strident] or [+strident] would not seem to be immediately useful because the basic articulatory productions go unspecified. Furthermore, it is difficult to assume that generalization training would be enhanced by classifying sounds as [+strident] or

---

[1]Features used here are defined as follows.

Stridency: Of the English fricatives /f, v, s, z, ʃ, ʒ/ are [+strident], and /θ, ð, h/ are [−strident]. The [+strident] sounds are characterized by considerable turbulence (noisiness) at the point of articulation.

Coronal: Sounds distinguished by the raising of the blade of the tongue from its neutral position. Apicals, dentals, and palatals are [+coronal]: /r, l, t, d, θ, ð, n, s, z, ʃ, ʒ, tʃ, dʒ/.

High: Sounds characterized with regard to the placement of the body of the tongue. Consonants marked as [+high] are /tʃ, dʒ, ʃ, ʒ, k, g, n/; those marked as [−high] are /r, l, p, b, f, v, m, t, d, θ, ð, n, s, z/.

[−strident]. Can we assume, for example, that /θ/ and /ð/ would be learned fairly easily, simply because the [−strident] consonants /t, d, n/ are correctly pronounced?

Consider now the anterior feature. This feature distinguishes between sounds produced along the anterior-posterior dimension: [+anterior] defines sounds produced forward of the production for /ʃ/, and [−anterior] includes sounds back of this position. Sounds marked as [+anterior] are: /l, p, b, f, v, m, t, d, θ, ð, n, s, z/.

The "feature" anterior varies with regard to place, manner, and voicing. To indicate that a single feature, such as anterior, is available, seems to have little relationship to the reality of articulatory productions. It is interesting to note, however, that children have no difficulty learning to understand and produce sounds that are forward of a particular point in the mouth. To them, the feature of anterior is very real.

Considering the findings of the bulk of the studies on articulatory inconsistency, I would regard the McReynolds and Huston conclusion, that features not produced in target sounds will appear in the productions of other sounds, an incontrovertible fact. Nevertheless, the Chomsky-Halle feature system may pose problems in interpretation for some features if statements about physiological capabilities are made.

It should be emphasized that the issue we are discussing may be misinterpreted along another dimension, that of the physiological capacity to produce a sound or set of sounds. Inferences about the capacity of a child to produce a "feature" are constrained by the particular feature system and by our willingness to accept certain abstractions. Even when we exclude Jakobsonian features, which in modern phonological theory do not have physiological reality, a certain degree of abstraction is involved.

To make this point clear, consider the manner feature of frication. Production of manner features, as we know, is not limited to one point in the mouth or vocal tract. Frication can occur at the teeth and lips (/f, v/), between the teeth (/θ,ð/) at the alveolar ridge (/s, z/), at the palate (/ʃ,ʒ/), and at the glottis (/h/). In languages other than English, frication has been observed to be produced at points not reflected by the set of English fricatives.

Now for the point we are trying to make. Can we regard manner features, such as frication, equivalent for different places of articulation? Can we say with certainty that frication at the alveolar ridge is equivalent to that produced between the teeth? Essentially the position I took in 1969 was that, within limits, this approach seems reasonable. The respiratory, laryngeal, and articulatory adjustments, necessary to produce frication, are similar throughout the vocal tract, so that we may rule out physiological insufficiencies when there is failure at one point of articulation and success at another point.

If, for example, a child without neurological involvement can produce /f, v, θ, ð, ʃ, ʒ/, but fails on /s, z/, is he capable of producing the manner feature of frication at the alveolar ridge? If the child produces no alveolar sounds (such as /n, d, t/) we might be hesitant to say yes. However, the fact that there are dental and palatal fricatives leads us to believe that alveolar fricatives can be made. If alveolar sounds /n, d, t/) can be produced, we would conclude that frication in the alveolar region should not be difficult to teach.

The above issue was not central to Walsh's reservations about the use of the Chomsky-Halle system for the type of research McReynolds and Huston conducted. His concern was more abstract. He felt that a single Jakobsonian feature could not adequately describe an articulatory production, and, therefore, generalizations regarding articulatory productions would be inappropriate.

Credit should be given to Walsh (1974) for noting that Jakobsonian features often lead to ambiguous and unclear interpretations regarding articulatory capacities. I am largely in agreement with Walsh, although he incorrectly concluded that I favored Jakobsonian features in the treatment of children with articulation disorders (Walsh, 1974, p. 38). I introduced Jakobsonian features in order to describe phonological acquisition. If Walsh had read further, he would have realized that I continued to recommend a phonetic based system for teaching articulatory productions.

Still there is another way in which distinctive features can be misused when applied to production segments. By definition, distinctive features are those elements designed to accommodate the phonological grammars of adult languages. For this reason, it is somewhat incorrect to use Jakobsonian features to describe the phonetic errors of young children. A distinctive feature is an abstract entity, bipolar in form, whose validity is established after careful and exhaustive research of the phonological grammars of a great number of languages.

Conceivably, phonological grammars can be developed for young children. An outcome of research on child phonology would be the establishment of a set of distinctive features that could be used in the same way distinctive features are used with adult grammars: as the basic elements of phonological rules. However, when features are used to assess the proportion of correct articulatory productions, then, by definition, phonological abstractions are not being studied.

It is therefore incorrect, in the strictest sense, to speak of "the percentage of correct distinctive features" because articulatory productions, not phonological abstractions, are of concern. A distinctive feature can be assigned only to a phonological grammar; it cannot be partially correct. The easiest way out of this definitional straightjacket is not to discard important data, but to recognize that the special vocabulary of a discipline has been violated.

Clinical Implications

There are instances in which Jakobsonian features may have an important if not direct relationship to the teaching of articulatory productions. We can illustrate this point by once again referring to the stridency feature. This feature was originally defined by Jakobson, Fant, and Halle (1952) in acoustical terms: [+strident] referred to sounds having irregular wave forms, giving the perceptual impression of noise, and [−strident] referred to sounds having regular wave forms, for which the impression of noise was less.

At times, it may be clinically important to consider features that are only indirectly related to articulatory productions. Let us assume that a child misarticulates strident fricatives (/s, z, ʃ, ʒ, f, v/) but correctly produces non-strident fricatives (/θ, ð/). This pattern of errors cannot be attributable to chance. A factor common to the [+strident] sounds must account for their consistent misarticulation. It is probably the acoustic similarity among the [+strident] fricatives that has caused difficulty for this child.

Articulatory training would involve teaching [−strident] frication as a substitute response for all six [+strident] fricatives. The noisy fricative might be an expirated snore, a velar fricative, or production of a modified /θ/, a forward blowing with the teeth closed. The six sounds would be trained as a group. For example, if training is begun with the expirated snore, denoted s̩ŋ (see Chapter 5), initial emphasis would be placed on mastering this sound. The clinician would pronounce each [+strident] fricative and ask the child to respond with his newly acquired expirated snore, as follows:

Clinician says	Child responds
/si/	/s̩ŋi/
/zi/	/s̩ŋi/
/θi/	/s̩ŋi/
/ði/	/s̩ŋi/
/ʃi/	/s̩ŋi/
/iʒ/	/s̩ŋi/

Gradually the s̩ŋ response would be shaped into a correct target fricative.

In this instance, the training program was governed by the observation that a group of incorrectly produced sounds all shared a common target feature specification. By emphasizing only production features in clinical practice, important relationships may go unnoticed.

Another point relating to the usefulness of Jakobsonian features needs to be considered. Pollack and Rees (1972) have suggested that difficulty in treatment may be related to the degree of difference in feature specifications between the target sound and the error sound. Let us call this the "off-target" hypothesis. As an example, /p/ substituted for /b/ would be regarded as a small degree of difference. A large degree of difference would be instanced by /θ/ substituted for /b/. In the p/b substitution only voicing is changed. The difference is much greater for the θ/b substitution, where voicing, manner, and place are changed.

Walsh's criticism pertains only to the fact that Pollack and Rees used Jakobsonian features to make their point. We recognize, of course, that Walsh's major purpose for writing his paper was to show that Jakobsonian features were not only misused but were unsuitable for describing articulatory errors. Nonetheless, I believe that all current feature systems would fail if the evaluation metric is a quantitative index. Walsh's discussion of this issue might leave the reader with the impression that the off-target hypothesis is poorly conceived. It is reasonable only if classes of sounds are considered separately (e.g., stops, fricative, and vowels). It does not work well across all sound types regardless of the feature system. In the pages ahead we make use of the principle provided by Pollack and Rees without doing damage to Walsh's position.

CLINICAL INSTRUCTION AND FEATURES

It now may be clear that there are essentially two ways in which features can be used in clinical instruction: a) as speech production segments that can be manipulated or varied directly by response modification procedures, and b) as higher order segments that are to be used in phonological descriptions of articulatory errors. We conclude this chapter by illustrating further these two properties of features.

Articulatory Errors

Segment Considerations   Articulatory errors can be described along several dimensions. Consider, for example, the physiological dimension.

We can describe in fairly complete detail the errors of production by making use of palatography or cineradiographic filming. Unfortunately, these instruments are not readily available to the practicing speech clinician. If they were, target positions as well as the dynamics of articulatory movements could be evaluated and correlated with perceptual (phonetic) judgments.

Perceptual judgments are reflected in phonetic transcriptions, where deviations from normal speech production are usually indicated by features, sounds, or both. For example, consider the following errors for the /s/ and /r/ sounds:

Target sound	Sound change	Feature change
/s/	/θ/	alveolar to interdental
/s/	/t/	frication to stop
/r/	/w/	retroflex alveolar to labial
/r/	/j/	retroflex alveolar to palatal

As shown above, the errors for /s/ and /r/ are described along two dimensions, sounds and features. For example, when /s/ is substituted by /θ/, the significant phonetic feature change is an interdental substitution for an alveolar position. Frication has been maintained, but place of articulation has been altered. To correct this /s/ error, placement rather than manner would need to be taught.

Phonetic transcription may give insights as to target positions, but knowledge of the actual articulatory movements, of course, would remain largely unknown. It remains to be determined, however, whether or not precise physiological information regarding transitional movements should be conveyed to a child or, for that matter, to an adult (see Chapter 6).

One unexplored method to teach transitional movements might be to develop a device that would enable the articulation-learner to track a visual image. An outline of the superior borders of the oral cavity as well as lingual movements might be displayed on a monitor. Errors in tracking could be indicated verbally or by pictorial display. When movements failed to match ideal movements, the discrepancy would be displayed on a screen.

Visual tracking has been used to teach pitch contours, vowels, and consonants to second language learners. Lane (1968) developed a procedure that enabled subjects to receive psychophysical feedback as they learned new pitch contours. Kalikow and Swets (1972) used complex electronic gear to teach English vowels and consonants (voice onset time and aspiration) to Spanish speakers. Their device displayed the subjects' targets relative to ideal targets. It remains to be determined whether feedback devices can be developed for displaying movements to and away from the target positions of sounds. As of now, visual feedback systems offer less precision than expert ears, which hear sounds not as isolated targets but as "syllabic" units—targets and transitional movements. Furthermore, as is discussed in Chapter 4, the proper kind of speech discrimination can facilitate the learning of speech production movements. Coincidentally, the electronic technology used to teach speech sound discrimination is relatively simple (Winitz, 1969).

Types of Articulatory Errors   A very fine summary of articulation errors is reported in Van Riper and Irwin (1958). Drawing from a number of research studies, Van Riper and Irwin (1958) summarized the common errors for speech sounds frequently found defective. We think these findings are of interest to the practicing speech pathologist, and, therefore, below are listed the errors, in order of frequency, for the /s/, consonantal /r/, /l/, /ʃ/, and /k/:

	/s/	/r/	/l/	/ʃ/	/k/
1.	[θ]	[w]	[w]	[tʃ]	[t]
2.	[l̥]²	[j]	[j]	[s]	[ʔ]
3.	[ʃ]	[ʁ]³	[hw]	[l̥]	[h]
4.	[t]	[v]	[ʌ]⁴	[s]	[tʃ]
5.	[f]	[f]	[r]	[ʒ]	[g]

In looking over the errors for each of the above sounds, a degree of consistency appears: The error sounds resemble the target sound in voicing, place, and manner of articulation. For example, [θ], a voiceless fricative, is generally found to replace /s/, another voiceless fricative. Similarly, the "semivowels" /r/ and /l/ are replaced by [w], also a semivowel.

Next, it is interesting to observe that, when the most frequent substitution for all five sounds is considered (the sounds assigned to number 1), the error is one of place. Manner of articulation (fricative, glide, or stop) is the same for the target sound as for the error substitution. As indicated above, /s/ and /ʃ/ are fricatives and are substituted by fricatives or affricates, and the semivowels /r/ and /l/ are substituted by /w/, also a semivowel. The /k/ is substituted by /t/, a stop (or plosive).

With few exceptions the voicing feature remains unchanged. If the target sound is voiced the error sound is voiced, and if the target sound is

---

²Voiceless [l].
³Back [r].
⁴Palatal [l].

voiceless the error sound is voiceless. Some manner changes can be observed to occur for relatively infrequent errors: /t/ for /s/, /hw/ for /l/, /tʃ/ for /k/, etc.

The above results are basically similar to those reported by Cairns and Williams in a study published in 1972. Compiling data from a large number of subjects from a midwestern community and reflecting the age range from first grade to high school, Cairns and Williams reported the most frequent error for four sounds:

/s/	/r/	/l/	/ʃ/	/k/
distortion	[w]	[w]	distortion	not included

Consistent with the findings of Van Riper and Irwin, the substitution errors were overwhelmingly a change in one specification of a feature. Furthermore, Cairns and Williams found that the errors were entirely unidirectional. Target sounds made with the front of the tongue (e.g., /r, l, s/) were substituted by sounds made at other points in the mouth, as well as by the front of the tongue, whereas sounds not produced by the front of the tongue (e.g., /f, p, k/) were substituted by sounds other than front-tongue sounds. These findings should be accepted with caution because Cairns and Williams included only the most frequent sound substitutions. In addition, the number of target sounds they studied was somewhat limited. A reexamination of the data provided by Van Riper and Irwin provides evidence that front-tongue sounds appear as substitutions for non-lingual sounds (e.g., /θ/ for /f/) and for velar sounds (e.g., /t/ for /k/), indicating that substitution errors are multidirectional with regard to place.

With regard to manner of articulation, Cairns and Williams (1972) found that continuants (fricatives, such as /f/ and /θ/) were substituted by stops, but the reverse was not found. However, Van Riper and Irwin (1958) reported that stops are substituted by fricatives, but that these substitutions are relatively infrequent.

The above discussion of error types would not have been possible without our tacit understanding of phonetic segments. By emphasizing feature alterations, rather than sound substitutions, as traditionally has been the custom, sophisticated hypotheses of the articulation learning process can be generated. We now turn to the role features play as elements in the phonological rules of children with articulation disorders.

Phonological Rules and Misarticulations

Consider the following example. A young child misarticulates postvocalic consonants, that is, words having shapes such as VC, CVC, CCVC, etc. On close examination the errors involve only the feature "stridency." All

[−strident] sounds become stops, [−continuant] in the nomenclature of modern phonological theory, and all [+strident] consonants are omitted. Represented by formula we can express the patterns of misarticulations as follows:

Rule 1:   [−*strident*] *becomes* [−*continuant*].
Rule 2:   [+*strident*] *becomes null after vowels*.

Changes governed by rule 1 would result in misarticulations of a number of sounds, including /r, l, θ, ð/. Place of articulation would not be altered, the stops being produced at the same general point in the oral cavity as the continuants. The /r/ would be substituted by a retroflex stop, the /l/ by a lateral stop, and the /θ/ and /ð/ by voiceless and voiced interdental stops, respectively.

Rule 1 does not specify subtle phonetic changes. Close observation might reveal that the dental stops, which replaced the /θ/ and /ð/, might be characterized by excessive aspiration. However, as shown later, precise phonetic transcription is not central to the issue under discussion.

Application of rule 2 would result in omissions of the following consonants when they occur following a vowel: /f, v, s, z, ʃ, ʒ, tʃ, dʒ/.

Perhaps some of the failures we experience in clinical practice can be attributed to the fact that isolated sounds rather than patterns of sounds are treated. Children may fail to generalize beyond that which they are taught because certain "natural" patterns of errors are ignored.

Is it not possible that increased efficiency in correcting the sound errors reflected in rules 1 and 2 might be gained by teaching the [−strident] sounds, /r, l, θ, ð/ as a group, before initiating training on the [+strident] sounds? The point that we have just raised pertains to generalization training, a topic to be considered in more detail later.

It is our belief, contrary to that held by Walsh, that articulatory training involves more than production training. Attention needs to be given to the organization of phonetic errors, which we hope can be described by phonological rules. To ignore this consideration would mean to focus on isolated production movements, a position that, historically, has been taken by most researchers in this discipline.

We now turn to a presentation of the phonological behavior of children with misarticulations, as reported by a few investigators. Halle (1964b), a leading theorist in the study of phonology, summarized in rule form the observations of Applegate (1961), who reported on the articulatory errors of a young child. The rules that Halle devised pertained to the following errors:

Glottal stop substitution		Other stop substitutions	
Standard word	*Child's pronuncia-tion*	*Standard word*	*Child's pronuncia-tion*
did	/dɪʔ/	does	/dʌd/
paper	/peɪʔ/	talks	/takt/
cake	/keɪʔ/	takes	/teɪkt/

In the first set of words, a glottal stop is substituted for /d, p, k/. In the second set of words, the /s, z/ sounds are substituted by stops. Halle's two rules were as follows (1964b, p. 343):

> (1) in a word containing several identical stop consonants, all but the first of these is replaced by a glottal stop.
> (2) all continuants are replaced by the cognate stops.

It would be of interest to speculate as to how one would go about the job of correcting the errors of this child. Assuming that this child's auditory discrimination is normal, my own preference would be to teach reduplication for the set of words in which ʔ /[+stop] substitution occurs, e.g., /dɪdɪ/, /peɪ peɪ/, and /keɪ keɪ/. When these productions are well established, I would transfer these new responses to the specific lexical items in which the errors occurred. Training would begin by placing the objects paper and cake in front of the child as he continues to produce reduplication. Gradually these reduplicated sequences would be faded from practice.

For the set of sounds marked by [+stop]/[+fricative] substitution, I would introduce in syllables a fricative form such as a bilabial fricative, blowing air through partially constricted lips. After this fricative production is stabilized, I would begin training on the /s/ and /z/ fricatives.

I am not convinced, as Walsh seems to be, that, for the kind of generalization training just described, the appropriate feature system, one which he has designed, is intuitively obvious, although it is difficult not to choose the system that generates preferred descriptions of phonological behavior. In fact, this issue is deserving of considerable research. In any event, it is clear that consideration of the phonological patterns of children with delayed articulation is an important dimension of the clinical process. The clinical routines need to reflect the pattern that seems to underlie each set of articulatory errors. Compton (1970, p. 328) recognized this issue well when he said, "... the errors characterizing articulatory disorders are generally not specific to single sounds but, rather, are a reflection of systematic patterns of errors encompassing entire classes of sounds possessing one or more features in common."

Another interesting investigation of phonological deviance was reported by Compton (1970). "Tom," the child studied in detail by

Compton, had a number of articulation errors. Not all of the errors are reported here, but the essence of Compton's observations is preserved.

The correct productions and/or substitutions for five word-initial consonants are listed below:

Standard sound	Correct productions	Errors
/ʃ/	/ʃ/	/s, k/
/s/	/s/	/k/
/tʃ/		/s, k/
/f/		/k/
/k/	/k/	

Compton recognized that the above set of errors reflected an underlying pattern of errors. He developed a set of rules to capture this fact.

The two rules presented below are modifications of Compton's rules. Jakobsonian features are used in place of the traditional place, manner, and voicing features. The rules are somewhat different from those given by Compton, yet there is a certain basic similarity. The striking fact is that the stridency feature emerges as central to the articulatory deviations.

Rule 3: *Voiceless strident sounds (/ʃ, tʃ/) marked as [−anterior] become [+anterior]:*

$$\begin{bmatrix} +\text{strident} \\ -\text{anterior} \\ -\text{voice} \end{bmatrix} \qquad \text{become} \qquad [+\text{anterior}]$$

/ʃ, tʃ/   become   /s/

Rule 4: *Voiceless strident sounds are articulated as voiceless velar stops:*

$$\begin{bmatrix} +\text{strident} \\ -\text{voice} \end{bmatrix} \qquad \text{become} \qquad \begin{bmatrix} -\text{strident} \\ -\text{continuant} \\ -\text{anterior} \\ -\text{coronal} \end{bmatrix}$$

/ʃ, tʃ, s, f/   become   /k/

In another case study Compton (1970) described the "errors" of "Jim," a youngster whose use of nasals departed considerably from the community norms. After thorough analysis, Compton recommended a program of treatment based on the rules he developed. First, let us examine the rules, and second, the results of treatment.

In the word-final position, Jim lengthened the nasal sounds, /m, n, ŋ/, and either added a homorganic stop, /b-p/, /t-d/, /k-g/, or omitted the nasals entirely. In stressed syllables the stop is [+voice], and in unstressed syllables it is [−voice].

The three errors for each of the three final nasals can be condensed by using braces:

Rule 5a: /m/ becomes $\begin{Bmatrix} \text{omitted ([}\phi\text{])} \\ \text{/m/ lengthened followed by /p/} \\ \quad \text{in unstressed syllables (/m:p/)} \\ \text{/m/ lengthened followed by /b/} \\ \quad \text{in stressed syllables (/m:b/)} \end{Bmatrix}$

Rule 5b: /n/ becomes $\begin{Bmatrix} \text{[}\phi\text{]} \\ \text{/n:t/ in unstressed syllables} \\ \text{/n:d/ in stressed syllables} \end{Bmatrix}$

Rule 5c: /ŋ/ becomes $\begin{Bmatrix} \text{[}\phi\text{]} \\ \text{/ŋ:k/ in unstressed syllables} \\ \text{/ŋ:g/ in stressed syllables} \end{Bmatrix}$

By using Jakobsonian features the rules for lengthening developed by Compton can be collapsed into the following rule:

Rule 6: $\begin{bmatrix} + \text{ nasal} \\ \alpha \text{ anterior} \\ \beta \text{ coronal} \end{bmatrix}$ becomes $\begin{bmatrix} + \text{ nasal} \\ + \text{ consonantal} \\ \alpha \text{ anterior} \\ \beta \text{ coronal} \\ + \text{ length} \end{bmatrix} \begin{bmatrix} - \text{ nasal} \\ + \text{ continuant} \\ \alpha \text{ anterior} \\ \beta \text{ coronal} \\ \gamma \text{ voice} \end{bmatrix}$ [γ stress]

The variables $\alpha, \beta,$ and γ serve to indicate that the value assigned to the feature can be either + or −. The value of the variable is the same (+ or −) throughout the rule. For example, for rule 6, the anterior, coronal, and stress features can be marked − or +. To indicate that /m/ (rule 5a) is lengthened followed by /p/ in unstressed syllables, we would have:

$\begin{bmatrix} + \text{ nasal} \\ + \text{ anterior} \\ - \text{ coronal} \end{bmatrix}$ becomes $\begin{bmatrix} + \text{ nasal} \\ + \text{ consonantal} \\ + \text{ anterior} \\ - \text{ coronal} \\ + \text{ length} \end{bmatrix} \begin{bmatrix} - \text{ nasal} \\ - \text{ continuant} \\ + \text{ anterior} \\ - \text{ coronal} \\ - \text{ voice} \end{bmatrix}$ [− stress]

After making the above analysis of Jim's errors, Compton devised a plan of treatment. According to Compton (1970, p. 335) "... the clinician worked individually with Jim on the production of final /m/, the goal being to eliminate the unusual lengthening of final nasals and the accompanying release into oral stops..." Nasals /n/ and /ŋ/ were not treated during this segment of the training program, which lasted five weeks.

Jim's retest scores indicated that /m/ was correctly articulated in final position, as one might well expect. The effect of training was not limited to /m/. Training had generalized across nasal sounds, a kind of confirmation of Compton's analysis of Jim's phonology of final nasals (rule 5).

As clinicians become skilled in writing rules, the approach taken by Compton should become more general. However, rule-writing will not become popular until there is firm recognition that articulation training encompasses more than the teaching of production gestures. Patterns of behavior are clearly involved.

SUMMARY

In summary, it can be said that articulation training is a complex process involving both the teaching of specific articulatory productions as well as teaching that leads to generalization.

Walsh, after making a number of important observations relative to the use of Jakobsonian features in treating articulatory disorders, finally concluded that only "language-specific articulation features" were of interest to speech pathologists.

In making this statement, Walsh viewed articulatory modification as entirely phonetic. It remains to be determined whether or not phonetically based feature systems will be adequate or appropriate for describing the abstract phonological generalizations of children with articulatory errors. As of now, it is difficult to see how generalizations can be made of articulatory defective systems, if language-specific features are used. Conceivably, rules might be developed for describing a systematic change in articulatory performance and yet involving a number of apparently diverse points of articulation.

There is the possibility that universal laws govern articulatory errors, and if so, certain generalizations might be lost by using narrowly language-specific (production) features (see Salus and Salus, 1974). Distinctive features have been used to compare linguistic growth across languages, and articulatory errors can be viewed within this same framework. We would not at this time discount the eventual usefulness of any particular feature system, because the important studies on articulatory generalization remain to be done.

Now that this rather lengthy chapter has been completed, we can move on to a consideration of the dimensions of articulatory training. Our first task is to examine articulatory proficiency.

CHAPTER 3

The Articulation Test: A First Look

Several years ago, I suggested that articulation tests were used in six different ways (Winitz, 1969). I still hold to my original cataloguing of articulation tests. At that time I indicated that they were used to: a) establish phonetic proficiency, b) screen, c) diagnose, d) predict, e) ascertain age of correct usage for individual sounds, and f) set up a program of instruction.

Without reviewing all of the evidence, it is now clear that articulation tests predict and diagnose very poorly. As a point of fact, their only reliable function is that of assessing phonetic proficiency, the results of which are used to index incorrect sound productions.

Perhaps in the not too distant future, articulation tests can be developed for providing information about the clinical process. As of now, the primary function of an articulation test is to determine sounds or patterns of sounds that need correction. Traditionally, words or pictures are used to elicit sounds. Tests vary in their composition; some are more complete than others. The clinician's task is clear. He or she is to listen to and record carefully the production of great numbers of sounds.

As of now, there is fairly good evidence to suggest that the production of sounds can be measured equally as well in isolated words as in sentences (see Winitz, 1969), as long as the phonetic environments are similar. However, when imitation is compared with spontaneous utterances, then imitative responses yield a higher percentage of correct responses whether or not the sound is tested in an isolated word or in conversation (Siegel, Winitz, and Conkey, 1963; Smith and Ainsworth, 1967; Faircloth and Faircloth, 1970). This point is discussed more fully in Chapter 8. In the meantime, the resolution of this issue seems unnecessary. Our first task should be to listen to our clients' conversational speech. Articulatory errors noted in conversational speech then can be examined in more detail. The articulation test should be a check for what we observe in conversational speech and not an independent measure.

ARTICULATION TEST PRINCIPLE 1

Children's articulatory errors should be examined initially in conversational speech. Errors then should be tested in greater detail, eliciting sounds by the use of pictures or by imitation.

Initially, error sounds should be examined in all three word positions, and in blends, in a fairly large number of words and short phrases. It is important to know the distribution of each articulation error. Only after we have carefully checked many contexts will we be able to ascertain the range of severity for each sound. If it is found that errors do not occur consistently in all of the many contexts tested, then it is clear that the sound can be produced. At this point, we can quickly dismiss "motorical insufficiency" as a cause for the error.

ARTICULATION TEST PRINCIPLE 2

Determine the consistency of articulation errors by examining the error sounds in a great number of contexts.

In 1959, Curtis and Hardy examined the production of /r/ allophones for a group of children with /r/ errors. Of the many phonetic contexts tested, /r/ was most correctly produced in the /pr/ cluster. Trailing in second place was /dr/. Almost all of the subjects (93%) produced a correct /r/ in at least one /consonant + r/ context. Curtis and Hardy also found that the /consonant + r/ context produced a great number of correct /r/ productions. The environments that were most productive were: /pr-dr-tr-str-br/. These contexts should be examined first when articulation testing is done.

The correct production of the /s/ sound also varies as a function of context. Zehel et al., 1972 reported that the /s/ was most often said correctly in the following contexts: /rs-sp-sk-st-sd-sæ-sʌ/.

One should not be restricted to word boundaries in searching for productive contexts. McDonald (1964) suggests examining unusual contexts that result from the uncommon juxtapositioning of words. Contexts for /r/ might be: ball + red (-lr-), buzz + road (-zr-), and bar + vent (-rv-). We can do the same for /s/: bush + saw (-ʃs-), glass + box (-sb), and grass + rug (-sr-).

ARTICULATION TEST PRINCIPLE 3

Search for contexts in which the error sound is said correctly. Once these contexts are established, they can provide a base for generalization to other contexts.

Some would question the validity of testing a great number of contexts when a simpler procedure is available. It is called *stimulability* and was introduced by Milisen in 1954. After a preliminary articulation test is given, Milisen suggests that children be given the opportunity to try their luck at imitating. The clinician produces those sounds that were missed in the articulation test and the child is asked "to try to say them correctly." In Milisen's terminology, sounds that can be imitated correctly are referred to as stimulable. It seems clear that, if a sound can be corrected in only a few trials, there is a high likelihood that it can be taught quickly. However, as discussed later, acquisition and habitual use are two different matters. A child who learns to imitate correctly may not necessarily acquire "carryover."

ARTICULATION TEST PRINCIPLE 4

Ask the child to imitate several correct productions of his error sounds. If he imitates correctly, there is no need for further detailed testing. If he fails, the examination of other phonetic contexts would seem to be in order.

What if we find that a child can neither imitate correctly nor produce the sound correctly in a great number of contexts? Our objective, then, would be to determine whether the phonetic (distinctive) features of the sounds in error are present.

Clinical Examples

If, for example, a young child consistently omits /p/ and /b/ but can articulate correctly nasals and non-labial stops, chances are he can learn to produce the labials within a short period of time. Let us illustrate this situation:

Articulation errors	*Correct sounds*
/p/ omitted	/m/ correctly used
/b/ omitted	/k/ correctly used
	/g/ correctly used
	/t/ correctly used
	/d/ correctly used

The features for /p/ are: a) voiceless, b) bilabial, and c) stop. /b/ is the voiced cognate of /p/.

We can now examine other sounds to determine whether these features are available. The voiceless feature occurs in /k/ and /t/, and the voiced feature in /g/ and /d/. The /m/ sound contains the bilabial feature. The stop or interrupted feature is part of the /k, g, t, d/ sounds. It is clear that this subject is physiologically capable of producing the features for the production of /p/ and /b/.

Another example might be helpful. A young child lisps, producing a /θ/ for /s/, and /ð/ for /z/. Digressing for the moment, it is instructive to note that there are many children who lisp on /s/, but not on /z/. If this is the case, then, the features for a good /s/ production are clearly available. Returning to our sample child, who produces frontal lisps for /s/ and /z/, we note the following:

Articulation errors	*Correct sounds*
θ/s	/t/ correctly used
ð/z	/d/ correctly used
	/f/ correctly used
	/v/ correctly used
	/ʃ/ correctly used
	/ʒ/ correctly used

Phonetic features of the /s/ sound are: a) voiceless, b) lingual-alveolar, and c) fricative. Phonetic features of the /z/ sound are: a) voiced, b) lingual-alveolar, and c) fricative.

The features lingual-alveolar and fricative are incorrectly used in this child's attempts to produce /s/ and /z/. However, these features are available in the child's record. Note that the lingual-alveolar feature is essential for the production of /t/ and /d/, and that the /f, v, ʃ, ʒ/ sounds are fricatives. There is no reason why this child should not be able to learn correct /s/ productions.

Several children with a great number of misarticulations were tested by McReynolds and Huston (1971), as discussed in Chapter 2. These children misarticulated many of the English phonemes. There is no question that they would be regarded as having a severe articulation disorder. Yet, when McReynolds and Huston completed their features analysis, most of the children were found to articulate the missing features in other sounds or in their error substitutions.

ARTICULATION TEST PRINCIPLE 5

If, after thorough testing of many phonetic contexts, <u>misarticulated sounds are not found to have been said correctly, a feature analysis should be made</u>. The features of correctly uttered sounds as well as the substitution of incorrectly produced sounds should be noted. If the features making up the standard sound are available in the child's repertoire of sounds, the progress for correction is good.

There is another reason why a feature analysis is useful. It assists in determining the underlying consistency of an articulation disorder. We would not proclaim that there is consistency to a child's articulation errors if we did not have preliminary evidence to indicate that this is so (Haas, 1963; Compton, 1970; Weber, 1970). If errors are consistent, can they be called errors? Consistency implies rule-governed behavior. An error implies a miscalculation or a mislearned response. Children's misarticulations can be called errors as long as we recognize that what is meant by error is a set of behaviors that is at variance with the community language.

Clinical Examples

A young child was found to omit /s/ preceding /p/, /t/, and /k/. She pronounced the following words without an /s/:

Word	Child's pronunciation
stove	/touv/
spoon	/pun/
skip	/kɪp/

When the clinician listened to the child, the above words seemed to begin with a /d/. The reason these initial stops are identified as voiced is because they lack aspiration, that little puff of air that follows initial voiceless stops in English.

The omission of /s/, however, is consistent because it occurs before all voiceless stops. We can derive this rule: /s/ appearing before voiceless stops is omitted; the voiceless stop, although an initial, remains unaspirated.

Another clinical example is given below:

Word	Child's response
fun	/pʌn/
soup	/tup/
thirsty	/t͡ɜ̃stɨ/
ship	/kɪp/
valentine	/bælɛntaɪn/
zoo	/du/
the	/dʌ/
measure	/mɛgɚ/

Quickly glancing at the above words, we may observe that the misarticulations reflect consistency. The rule is: Fricatives become stops. The change from fricative to stop alters neither place of articulation nor voicing. The front fricatives /s, θ/ and /z, ð/ are replaced by the front stops /t/ and /d/, respectively. In the case of the two palatal fricatives, /ʃ/ and /ʒ/, their respective substitutions are /k/ and /g/.

ARTICULATION TEST PRINCIPLE 6

Examine a child's articulatory errors for consistency. See if you can describe the errors in terms of one or two phonetic features.

What is the rule for the following misarticulations?

Word	Child's response
cap, cab	/kæm/
coat, code	/koun/
back, bag	/bæŋ/

It is easy to see that the rule is: Final stops become nasals, and the nasal sound assumes the same place of articulation as the stop. It is important to realize that we are able to derive rules that pertain to more than one sound error because we employ features rather than sounds to describe articulatory errors.

When we use rules to describe articulatory deviations, it is not always clear whether the problem is one of discrimination or production. Let us assume we have discovered the rule that stops became nasal in the final position. It seems clear that place of articulation can be discriminated because the nasal errors retain the place of the stops. We do not know, however, whether the voiceless stops can be discriminated from the voiced stops nor whether nasals can be discriminated from oral stops. We would like to have this information before we begin our training program. The next chapter directly deals with discrimination training procedures, and so it is unnecessary to expand on this topic here. However, as shown later, we need to make a distinction between discrimination and conceptualization.

Before we conclude our discussion, it should be pointed out that we have neglected to emphasize two traditional purposes of articulation testing: prediction, and developmental maturity.

Predictive tests of articulation (Winitz, 1969) aim to assess articulatory performance at some later date. These tests are highly unreliable, and for this reason we do not recommend them. It seems that one cannot predict articulatory performance six months or one year later because the most important ingredient is usually left unmeasured. It is the relationship between the child and his environment. This critical component seems to be difficult to assess by standard testing procedures.

Tests of developmental maturity (see Templin, 1957) are, in essence, predictive tests. The purported purpose of these tests is to determine the average age at which each sound is correctly produced. When using developmental tests, clinicians not only compare a child's performance with his peers, but they make predictions about a child's performance at a later time. In this way developmental tests serve the same function as predictive tests.

Clinical Examples

Clinicians who opt to begin speech training because a sound is late in appearing are guided by the criterion of prediction. Assume that a child is five years old and he misarticulates /g/. According to norms provided by Templin (1957), the /g/ sound is mastered by four-year-old children. Correction would seem to be in order. The decision to correct, as we see it, is one of prediction because it is assumed that the sound will not be self-corrected in the near future.

When a child is brought to a speech clinic because he has not mastered one or more sounds, the issue of prediction reasserts itself. Let us assume that the mother of a five-year-old child is concerned that her child incorrectly articulates the /θ/ and /z/ sounds. The clinician agrees that these sounds are not said correctly, but indicates that the average child does not master them until age six. So child and mother are sent away and are told to return one year later if the sound errors are retained.

The clinician is betting that the /θ/ and /z/ will be acquired within a year; a prediction is being made. He or she is assuming that the child will follow his peers and self-correct his two sound errors; and if no progress is made, the child can be enrolled in the clinic at the proper age—an easy but unscientific solution.

We disagree with this approach. Speech training could have been accomplished just as easily a year sooner, and perhaps in a short period of time. Also, the concerns of the parent would have been allayed. Sometimes parental counseling can be helpful; the speech pathologist can advise the parent about speech errors, including important information on the onset and treatment of articulation errors. Often, however, parents who are overly concerned about their child's speech errors take advice poorly; frequently they do not remember what they are told. They may continue to relate to their child in a way that increases the severity of the disorder.

Using developmental norms as a guide for the time of correction involves a basic misconception about the articulatory learning process. Learning to articulate is a single process, whether carried out under highly controlled routines in the clinic or under the more haphazard conditions of the home. To be sure, we can speed the process of articulatory acquisition in the clinic, but the basic process by which sounds are acquired is no different in the clinic than in the home. This last statement should not be interpreted to mean that parents use the same techniques that clinicians use in treating children for whom an articulation error has stabilized; but only that the processes of acquisition—the perception, storing, and recalling of stimuli—are fundamentally the same. Furthermore, as indicated in Chapter 1, there are circumstances that inhibit, slow, or prevent language from developing. The correlation we have made between clinical instruction and normal language growth pertains, of course, only to situations that do not result in articulation errors.

If a clinician is unwilling to correct sounds because they appear late, according to developmental norms, and assumes that the sounds will change as a function of time, he is acting as though there were two acquisition processes, one in the home and one in the clinic. In fact, there is only one acquisition process. The controlling consequences begin as early as one year and essentially remain the same, although standards of excellence change, until about five years of age. Beyond that time, some parents become more stringent, perhaps delaying acquisition because they strive for perfection (see Winitz, 1969).

ARTICULATION TEST PRINCIPLE 7

Developmental tests should not be used for predictive purposes. They should be used as a guide for counseling parents. If a parent wants his child to be admitted to speech training because he is alarmed about the child's speech progress, our recommendation would be to treat the child.

Few parents seek clinical advice before their child's fifth birthday. However, if a child of three, for example, is totally unintelligible, parents often become alarmed. Chances are that concerned parents may inhibit the normal development of their child's speech, if they are not properly counseled. There is no better way to instruct a parent than to have him observe good language instruction practices (see Sommers, 1962).

A child of three, who has more misarticulations than is considered normal, should be treated. The treatment, as we see in the next chapter, should be shared by the parent and the clinician. If it is properly handled, one can accomplish a great deal with three-year-old children. In fact, six months of training at age three might reduce the need for training at a later time.

Again, there is no reason to believe that training in the clinic is in any way different from the language-teaching practices of the average parent. To be sure, a small proportion of mothers and fathers violate the practices we adhere to in the clinic (see Winitz, 1969), but the majority of parents do not. Parents provide children with enormous amounts of discrimination long before they begin to speak. Once children show signs of speaking, parents continually encourage them. Parents do not, of course, request that words be repeated, that the tongue should take a certain position in the mouth, or that the movements of front sounds be observed in the mirror. Yet parents unknowingly monitor their children's speech. Their children repeat words not because they are asked to, but because it is part of the communicative interchange between parent and child.

Requests, commands, declarations, and commentary are the motivational elements on which good communication is built. Over time, incorrect articulatory responses are extinguished because the child's skill in discrimination increases, and the child's unintelligible articulatory patterns are misunderstood by the parent. It is not uncommon to hear parents use fragmented sentences in order to isolate what they regard as the source of the error. We hear parents say, "Not tomato—potato"—a short lesson in discrimination. We also know that parents respond to a child's utterances, such as "Give me the poon," with a request to repeat—"What do you want?"—followed by "Oh, you mean spoon."

In summary, then, we regard clinical speech practices and parental language instruction as practiced in the majority of homes to be one and the same. We know that serious language instruction is begun by the mother at about the time the child celebrates his first birthday. For this reason, we see no harm in practicing speech correction at an early age.

At this time, it is important to mention (see Winitz, 1969) that articulatory development beyond three years of age does not reflect a maturational component. By age three, children without organic deficiencies are capable of producing all of the phonetic features essential for the phonemes of the community language. Beyond then, articulatory growth reflects generalization of speech sounds to a large number of words, phonetic contexts, and grammatical components. Learning to articulate a sound correctly in all of its many and varied environments simply cannot be accomplished quickly.

CHAPTER 4

Discrimination Training and Auditory Practice

One reason adults may have difficulty discriminating between speech sounds is because their linguistic experience has been limited. For example, English speakers do not find it easy to distinguish among the three Malayalam /t/ sounds. Citizens of Southern India have no difficulty because these *t*'s must be perceived if words containing them are to be understood.

In Malayalam, speakers use a dental *t,* an alveolar *t,* and a postalveolar *t* (Catford and Ladefoged, 1968), as instanced in the following words:

Dental	*Alveolar*	*Postalveolar*
/muṭṭu/	/muttu/	/muṭṭu/
(pearl)	(density)	(knee)

With continued exposure and use, the young Southern Indian child learns to distinguish among these three *t's,* and thus has no difficulty distinguishing among the words for pearl, density, and knee.

There is some evidence to suggest that exposure may not be as critical as was previously assumed. Infants of about six weeks of age were found by Eimas et al. (1971) to be able to distinguish voiced-voiceless contrasts. In their study, the time between the release of the stop consonant and the beginning of voicing in the vowel was varied. This metric is called voice onset time (VOT). Linguistic investigations (Lisker and Abramson, 1964) have indicated that VOT, the temporal relation between the onset of laryngeal pulsing and supraglottal acoustic features, distinguishes between voiced and unvoiced initial stops. Furthermore, when many languages are considered, not all values of VOT are used. VOT values seem to cluster around several universal language points. The infants in the study of Eimas and his colleagues distinguished best between VOT's that are generally common to a great number of languages, suggesting that some distinctions may be innate.

On the other hand, we know from studies on the development of speech discrimination that many distinctions are not mastered until long after children have begun to talk (Winitz, 1969). Sounds that are acoustically close (Abbs and Minifie, 1969), or are smeared in running speech, may be causes for difficulty. Furthermore, because children have a need to communicate, they begin to utter words before all phonetic segments have been acquired. Judging from my experience with children and with adults learning a second language, a word is often produced incorrectly when there has been limited exposure. Say aloud the following Hebrew words three times. Then wait a few minutes and try to recall them. They are: /matate/ (broom), /iparon/ (pencil), /ʃemeʃ/ (sun). Chances are that you will be unable to recall the above words correctly. As a rule young children mispronounce their early words. With time, they change their incorrect productions to correct productions (Bullowa, Jones, and Duckert, 1964).

It is believed that habitual use of an incorrect sound obscures perceptual differences. I have suggested (Winitz, 1969), for example, that when a child has a history of a /w/ for /r/ substitution, discrimination between these sounds will be very difficult.

TESTING FOR SOUND DISCRIMINATION

Whatever the reason, children often have difficulty hearing distinctions between sounds. The research literature has demonstrated that children with speech errors evince considerably more discrimination errors than normal speaking children. There is, as indicated above, a fairly high relationship between speech discrimination and articulation. A child who does not hear differences between sounds hardly can be expected to produce sounds precisely. It seems reasonable, then, to test for the discrimination of only those sounds that are in error. We do not recommend testing speech sounds that are not in error. It is necessary, then, to make up a discrimination test for each of the children or adults whom you test. A general discrimination test, such as the Wepman Auditory Discrimination Test (Wepman, 1958), does not provide this kind of information. It may not, for example, include those sounds with which an individual child has difficulty.

Clinical Example

A young child substitutes the /w/ for the consonantal /r/ in initial word positions. Prepare a list of minimal pairs, as follows (asterisks indicate non-English words):

read	-	weed
rat	-	wat*
run	-	one
roast	-	woast*
right	-	white
ri*	-	wi*

The list should be more extensive than this sample one.

The testing can be done in two ways. In the traditional approach, same-different pairs are presented, such as: road-road, road-woad, and woad-woad. Here ask the child to determine whether each pair of words is the same or different.

Another procedure is to present only one word at a time. Ask the child to raise his hand when the word is correctly spoken. Here it is best to place a picture of the item before the child. Let him look at the picture first, before you produce the test word. Present in a random way correct and incorrect words for each picture.

If a child scores well (perhaps above 80%) you can be fairly certain that he can distinguish between /r/ and /w/. If the child discriminates some /r-w/ pairs, but not others, retest all pairs several more times to determine the consistency of the child's discriminations. It is very possible that he may distinguish between word:non-word pairs (rat-wat) but not between word:word pairs (read-weed) (Sapir, 1972). If so, it may suggest that his difficulty in discrimination may be acquired; he has learned not to discriminate between words. Also, the client may distinguish between non-word pairs, such as /ri-wi/, but not between word pairs, such as read-weed. If so, it would also suggest that phonetic discriminations are affected by lexical context. It is important to discover the contexts as well as the sounds that cause difficulty in discrimination. Once the source of difficulty is discovered, a level of training can be established.

SOUND DISCRIMINATION PRINCIPLE 1

Test for specific discrimination errors and try to determine the linguistic environments in which the errors occur.

Clinical Example

The clinician's initial impression is that the client in question substitutes an initial /t/ for /k/. The substitution occurs when /k/ precedes the front vowels /i/ and /ɪ/. In other instances, the /t/ for /k/ substitution does not occur. A close phonetic analysis reveals that the /t/ substituted for /k/ is not alveolar. Rather, the sound is a very forward /k/. The central part of the tongue makes contact with the palate. Discrimination training between /k/ and /t/, such as ki-ti or kip-tip, is unrelated to the specific sound substitution. Training should involve discrimination between the error sound, as the child produces it, and the correct sound. To be able to simulate the child's errors, it is necessary to listen to and practice the child's error production many times.

SOUND DISCRIMINATION PRINCIPLE 2

Train clients to discriminate between their sound error and the standard pronunciation.

The question is often asked whether discrimination training will result in correct production without any speech training. There is some preliminary evidence (Winitz, 1969) to suggest that it will, but only under certain circumstances (Winitz and Bellerose, 1967). At this time, it is best to suggest that discrimination training will affect changes in production if: a) the production features are in the individual's repertoire, and b) the training is extensive and carefully carried out.

Clinical Example

A young child incorrectly produces /θ/ for /s/. The child, however, correctly produces /z/. It is clear, then, that the phonetic (distinctive) features of /s/ are currently being produced by the child. A segment of the child's articulation test reveals the following:

θ/s
/k/ correctly used
/t/ correctly used
/z/ correctly used

The /s/ is a voiceless apicoalveolar fricative; that is, the apex or forward part of the tongue makes contact with the alveolar ridge. The /z/ is, as we know, a voiced apicoalveolar fricative. The /s/ and /z/ are made in essentially the same way, with the exception of the voice feature.

The feature of unvoicing appears in this child's record, since his articulation test shows that /t/, /k/, and several other voiceless sounds are correct. Furthermore, unvoicing occurs in /θ/, his substitution for /s/, indicating again that unvoicing can be produced.

The fact that all the features essential for the production of /s/ are within the capabilities of this child would seem to indicate that the correct production of /s/ probably would occur as a result of intensive discrimination training (Winitz and Preisler, 1965). By intensive discrimination training, we mean sufficient training trials so that a strong auditory image is developed.

SOUND DISCRIMINATION PRINCIPLE 3

Discrimination training may affect changes in production if the features essential for the sound(s) in question are currently in the productive repertoire of the client.

How is discrimination training carried out? It can be done in a highly controlled situation, as indicated above. By a controlled situation, we mean one in which the clinician sits near the child and drills on phonetic contrasts.

There is a more "natural" way to teach sound discriminations. We know from studies on the acquisition of child language (reviewed by Winitz and Reeds, 1975), that children are encouraged by their mothers to listen before they are asked to speak. In fact, mothers rarely correct their children's speech, and when they do their children have essentially mastered their native language. Corrections are generally limited to obscenities, incorrect verb usage (such as "he swung" for "he swinged"), and descriptive niceties (such as ''Johnny and I'' for ''me and Johnny''). In a word, parents accept what their children say.

Why, you may ask, do children change their articulations if their parents do not correct them? An eleven-month-old girl studied by Bullowa, Jones, and Duckert (1964) was observed to utter /tu/ for *shoe*. At twelve months she changed her pronunciation to /tʃu/, and between this time and seventeen months /tsu/ was heard. By the end of the seventeenth month /ʃu/ was uttered most of the time. The progression from /tu/ to /ʃu/ took six months, an interval we cannot regard as short.

Why did she change her pronunciation? We can only guess that this child, like so many others reported in the literature, perfected her articulation because her environment demanded change. Our conjecture is that an incorrect pronunciation will be misinterpreted by a child's mother, father, or any other person with whom the child interacts. The early pronunciations of ''shoe'' easily could have been confused with a great number of other words. When there is misinterpretation, a child will listen more carefully and try to correct his pronunciations.

Support for our position is admittedly slim (see Chapter 1). Yet I have observed many instances of misunderstanding in my contact with young children. Most recently, a young child asked me to give her /freʃmɪnts/ from a table filled with all sorts of wonderful looking desserts. After carefully examining the entire table, I said there were no mints. Her mother, standing nearby, overheard our conversation and said that her daughter was asking for *refreshments*.

Most importantly, it has been shown by Brown and his colleagues (see Brown, Cazden, and Bellugi, 1969) that correction of articulations or the approval of correct productions are uncommon practices of mothers. Apparently, parents do not correct their children's speech. They do not ask their children ''to say the word over,'' ''repeat after me,'' or ''listen and try and say it the right way.'' Rather, parents respond inappropriately or incorrectly to a word or sentence which they do not understand. To a child, an inappropriate response by a parent leads to bewilderment and confusion. As a result, children listen more attentively and make every attempt to modify their articulations.

We can now propose another way to teach speech sound discriminations. It is an approach that more closely parallels normal speech development. It is also simple to do, but it means shaking yourself loose from the traditional practice of emphasizing production.

The general procedures are as follows:

1. Determine those sounds and contexts with which your client has difficulty.

2. Prepare and gather objects in which these sounds are used.
3. Develop activities that thoroughly entertain and involve your client.
4. Repeat many times the names of the objects.

5. When your client asks for an item, only give it to him when he says the object's name correctly. If he says it incorrectly, hesitate for a moment and sometimes give him the wrong item.

If, for example, your child substitutes /θ/ for /s/, gather items that begin with /s/ and /θ/ sounds. The /θ/ is an infrequent sound in English, complicating the training somewhat. You may have to invent names for animals like /θup/ and /θoʊldʒɚ/ to contrast with /sup/ and /soʊldʒɚ/.

As you engage the child in play activities, make him constantly responsible for selecting one of two items. Eventually he will learn to discriminate correctly. At the same time, the child will pester you to give him these objects. If he asks for /θoʊldʒɚ/, and it is obvious he wants the toy soldier, wait five seconds, then say, "OK, here it is," and hand him a different object, perhaps a toy lion. He will probably say that is not what he wanted. Then say, "OK, you meant 'soldier' not '/θoʊldʒɚ/.' You wanted the soldier; well here it is, take the soldier, and put the soldier here." With more training the child might even correct himself.

SOUND DISCRIMINATION PRINCIPLE 4

Actively engage the child in discrimination training by preparing interesting materials. Frequently contrast correct and incorrect productions. When the child incorrectly articulates, wait a few seconds, then respond inappropriately. Finally, respond appropriately by saying the name of the object several times before handing it to the child. As training continues, wait for the child to correct himself after you have responded inappropriately.

Everyone faces tough cases. So do not be surprised if you find children who fail to discriminate between sounds. Fortunately, we have procedures that can be used to teach difficult discriminations. The principle is very simple. Sound units that seem to be different—that is, whose phonemes show little overlap in features—are presented first. Gradually, the similarity between items is increased until the items look almost alike, in the case of visual stimuli, or almost sound alike, in the case of auditory stimuli.

Stimuli are similar, if they differ on only one or two dimensions. The sounds /p/ and /b/, which differ on the voicing dimension, are more similar than /p/ and /z/, which differ on three dimensions, namely, voicing, continuacy, and place of articulation.

The following two symbols look very much alike. In fact, you will have difficulty determining how they are different:

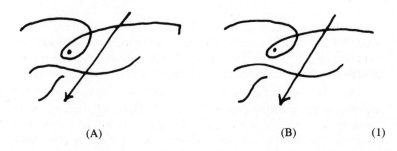

(A)   (B)   (1)

Now let us see how one can teach differentiation of these two visual displays so that children can learn without difficulty. The important distinction between these two symbols is presented on the first comparison so that the subject can focus on it. Watch the next three displays:

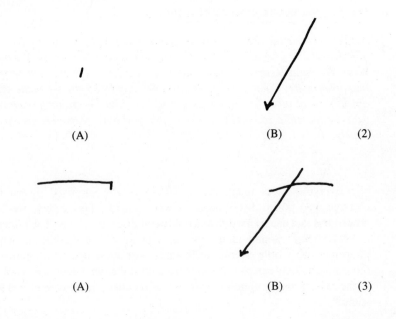

(A)   (B)   (2)

(A)   (B)   (3)

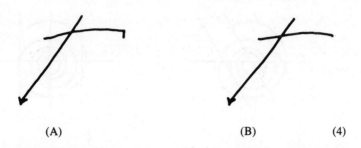

(A)   (B)   (4)

Now, the two displays can easily be discriminated, since the small vertical line in (A) was made clear from the beginning. Look back at the first pair (item 1). It is easy to distinguish between them because we know on what to focus.

If we use speech sounds, the discrimination training sequence cannot be fragmented in the above fashion. It may be possible, in some cases, with machine-produced speech, but obviously not practical. We can accomplish almost as much if we use the full range of English speech sounds.

In (5) below, we have two patterns, A and B, which are very different. In (6) they are somewhat similar, and in (7) they are almost identical:

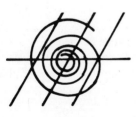
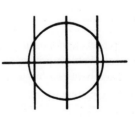

(A)   (B)   (5)

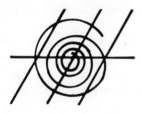
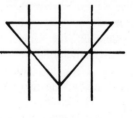

(A)   (B)   (6)

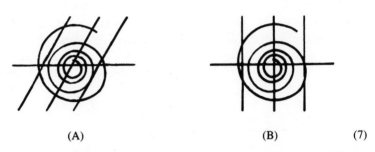

(A)   (B)   (7)

The only difference between the figures in (7) is that (A) has slanted lines, and (B) has vertical lines. In (5) we discriminate between triangle and spiral, in (6) between circle and spiral, and in (7) between slanted lines and straight lines. The lines are not the focus of attention in (5). However, the fact that the geometric forms of (7) can be easily distinguished is because the spiral is brought to our attention first, and   regarded   as irrelevant. In (6) the lines are not as easy to discriminate as the geometric forms are, yet we are able to notice them because the spiral-circle distinction is so easy that our attention can be directed elsewhere. In (7) we can no longer distinguish (A) and (B) on the basis of geometric form, and so we turn to a feature that we had noticed before but which was never distinctive. That feature is, of course, the vertical placement of the lines. In a sense, the sequence (5) (6), and (7) permits us to focus on the relevant dimensions because we learn what to focus on. Stated simply, we are taught what to look for.

Essentially the same procedures are followed in teaching difficult speech discriminations. We initially present sound contrasts that are easy to discriminate. As the sequence progresses, contrastive similarity is increased. Finally, the two sounds with which the child has difficulty are presented. The child will have little difficulty learning to discriminate between the relevant dimensions, because at this time all other dimensions can be easily discriminated and, thus, regarded as irrelevant.

Clinical Examples

A young child cannot easily discriminate between /w/ and /r/. The clinician decides to develop a program of instruction to assist the child in learning to discriminate between /w/ and /r/. The programmed sequence of phonemic contrasts is as follows:

1. /wa - ka/
2. /wa - ta/
3. /wa - ja/
4. /wa - ra/

There is preliminary evidence to show that a sequence similar to this can be used to teach the /r-w/ contrast (Winitz and Bellerose, 1967).

Let us consider a child who substitutes a lateral lisp for /s/. A suggested sequence for the lateral lisp, the voiceless fricative l (denoted [ɬ]) is as follows:

1. /ɬa - ka/
2. /ɬa - ta/
3. /ɬa - za/
4. /ɬa - sa/

If a child substitutes /θ/ for /s/, a proposed sequence might be:

1. /θa - wa/
2. /θa - da/
3. /θa - ta/
4. /θa - sa/

The discrimination training program is easy to administer. The first pair is presented several times, perhaps for an entire clinical session, until the child's level of correct responding is close to 80 to 90%. Then, begin teaching the second pair, and so on.

It is not necessary to teach only one vowel context; several can be used simultaneously. For example, you can teach /θa-wa/, /θi-wi/, and /θu-wu/, all at one time.

Creativity should not be abandoned in teaching sound discriminations. Assign puppets the names of each discrimination pair or command the children to jump when they hear one of the two pairs.

SOUND DISCRIMINATION PRINCIPLE 5

Difficult sound discriminations can be taught by developing a sequence of pairs in which phonetic differences are carefully programmed. The phonetic distance between early pairs should be very large. Gradually the phonetic distance should be narrowed.

Perhaps you noticed something unusual about the three programmed sequences in the clinical examples above. The first pair always begins with a syllable reflecting the error substitution: [w], [ɬ], or [θ]. The decision to begin with the error sound was predicated on an experiment reported in Winitz (1969). It was found that beginning with the correct or standard sound, such as /r/ rather than /w/, would fail to teach discriminations.

Let us see why we should begin with the error sound. A young child who has difficulty discriminating the printed *b* from *d,* and who always writes *b* for both sounds, would benefit from a programmed sequence if it began with *d*. Consider the following program for teaching the *b-d* discrimination:

$$
\begin{array}{ll}
1. & \text{d \quad o} \\
2. & \text{d \quad p} \\
3. & \text{d \quad b}
\end{array}
\tag{8}
$$

With this sequence, learning would be impaired because the sounds in the third pair would appear equivalent. Let us see why this would be so.

The child sees *d* and *b* but consistently writes *b*. We can diagram this process as follows:

Printed stimulus　　　　　*Implicit perception*　　　　　*Child's response*

d
b ———————————→ b – – – – – → b ———————————→ b

The above diagram means that, if either *d* or *b* is presented to the child, the implicit perception is always *b* and the overt response is always *b*. In the case of the first pair in (8), the child identifies *d* as *b*, since *b* is his implicit perception. In the second and third pairs the child continues to identify *d* as *b*. When the child sees the third pair, both *b* and *d* are perceived as *b*. In summary, the programmed sequence of (8) encourages the child to maintain a single implicit perception for *b* and *d*.

Now let us alter (8) to read as follows:

$$
\begin{array}{ll}
1. & \text{b \quad o} \\
2. & \text{b \quad q} \\
3. & \text{b \quad d}
\end{array}
\tag{9}
$$

In this program, the implicit stimulus *b* matches *b*, one of the printed letters for the first pair. Here, the printed letter and the implicit perception are identical. In the second pair (*b-q*) the implicit perception matches the printed letter *b*, and *b* must be distinguished from *q*. Because *b* and *q* are different, this discrimination can be made easily. Furthermore, the non-stem portions of *b* and *q* face opposite directions. This distinction will be noticed by the child, as it will be for *d-p*, the second pair in (8). However, for this second pair in (9), the difference will not only be noted, but the constancy between the implicit perception and *b* will continue to be maintained.

We can diagram the relationships thus far:

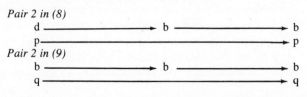

When pair 3 is presented, there will be generalization of the letters from pair 2 as follows:

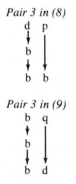

Pair 3 in (8)

Pair 3 in (9)

In (8) discrimination of the letters of the second pair, *d* and *p*, can be made because the implicit stimulus *b* differs from *p*. In (9) the discrimination of the second pair, *b* and *q*, also involves an implicit stimulus for *b*, but here the letter of the implicit stimulus *b*, and the physical stimulus, *b*, are identical. When the third pair of (9) is presented, *b* elicits *b* as expected, but *b* will be distinguished from *d* because the distinctive qualities of *q* will generalize to *d*. In the case of (8) *d* elicits the internal representation *b*, which, as we know, has been maintained throughout training. The distinctive qualities of *p* will generalize to *b*, and not to *d*, resulting in two stimuli, *b* and *d*, which are perceived as *b*.

SOUND DISCRIMINATION PRINCIPLE 6

Discrimination programs containing sequenced pairs will achieve little success unless the child's error responses are carefully considered. After the error responses are identified, they should appear early in the training sequence. The correct or standard sound should appear late in the programmed sequence.

Every effort should be made to present the sequence of programmed materials in a creative way. If, for example, a young child substitutes [ɬ] for /s/, several items should be introduced that begin with the [ɬ] sound. One can invent nonsense figures like the ones below:

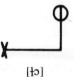

[ɬak]   [ɬɔ]   [ɬʌn]

The [ɬak] is contrasted with "sock," the [ɬ] with "saw," and the [ɬʌn] with "sun." Do not encourage the child to say these nonsense items, but there is no real harm if he does. Develop games in which the child is forced to make discriminations. You might ask him to jump over the item you name. Or he can be asked to tape the correct item to a window, or give it to another child. If you prefer, the items can be used in spinning games or matching games.

Do not be concerned that incorrect pronunciation in discrimination activities may generalize to production. Only nonsense items are used, and discrimination, not production, is being trained.

In time, the length of the unit is expanded. Contrastive expressions, such as "I see the wing on the table" and "I see the ring on the table" will develop focusing. Children will focus on the correct-incorrect contrast if the critical item cannot be identified from context. For the sentences, "The man thinks about his boy" and "The ship sinks quickly," a child would have little difficulty in identifying the contrast between "thinks" and "sinks." For the sentence pair, "The man examines the thumb" and "The man examines the sum," contextual cues are not available. Neither are they for the phrases "The boy sat glued" (a boy sitting in a chair watching television) and "The boy that glued" (a boy pasting pictures with glue). Another contrasting pair for /θ/ and /s/ is "surround the house" and "the round house." With a little imagination, many appropriate sentences and pictures can be developed.

With some sounds it is easy to develop sentential contrasts. For /k/ and /t/ we might have, "The lady carries the key in her hand" and "The lady carries the tea in her hand." A contrast involving /l/ and the omission of /l/ is "The man was unhappy about the fight" and "The man was unhappy about the flight."

SOUND DISCRIMINATION PRINCIPLE 7

Subsequent to the discrimination of isolated sound units, there should be emphasis on the discrimination of sounds in running speech.

We are now faced with an interesting question. Should discrimination training begin with isolated contrasts and proceed to sentences without intervening practice in production? This is a difficult question to answer; however, a point of view will be offered.

About midway in this chapter, we discussed the effect of discrimination training on production, concluding that discrimination training is most effective when the distinctive features appear in a child's record, even though they may be inappropriately used. For example, a child who substitutes /θ/ for /s/, but is found to substitute /t/ for /k/, most likely would learn to produce /s/ after discrimination training. The reason is that the lingual-alveolar feature is found in /t/.

In the child's verbal environment, as well as in the clinic, the standard (non-defective) pronunciations are used countless times, and most always in sentences. When a child learns to discriminate the standard sound from his substitution in sentences, he is then able to derive full benefit from his discrimination training because the contrasts outside of the clinic are primarily those that occur in running speech. It seems logical, then, to train the child to this point as quickly as possible. Furthermore, if the discrimination training is carried out in the matter suggested above—delay in responding, inappropriate responding, and repeated pronunciations on the part of the clinician, teacher, or parent—changes in production may result without the need for direct articulation training.

SOUND DISCRIMINATION PRINCIPLE 8

Because the standard sound occurs countless times in running speech, it is most logical to train a child to observe these contrasts as quickly as possible. Training in speech production should not begin until discrimination can be made easily between the standard and the non-standard sound in sentences. Thus, not until a high degree of discrimination training is achieved, would articulatory training begin.

Time and time again we hear the question: With which sound do we begin treatment? The answer to this question might be: Do not look at sounds, look at patterns of sounds.

Let us return to the child, described in Chapter 3, who omitted /s/ before voiceless stops, having errors and correct sounds as follows:

Response	Word
/pul/	spool
/tɪl/	still
/keɪt/	skate
/sup/	soup
/kɪs/	kiss

There is one unifying rule to describe the errors: /s/ is omitted before voiceless stops, but not elsewhere.

Additional study of this child reveals that there is good discrimination. Therefore, we may conclude that the /s/ omissions reflect conceptualization errors. The rule that certain words begin with two consonants, when the /s/ is involved, apparently has not been learned. It seems to be a question of conceptualization, not discrimination.

Clinical Examples

Using a procedure developed by LaRiviere et al. (1974), conceptualization can be taught by using a sorting task. The student hears a series of words or syllables and is asked to group each item into one of two categories by raising his right or left hand. The procedure is depicted as follows:

Stimulus	Raise left hand	Raise right hand
spool	✓	
pill		✓
Kate		✓
stick	✓	
pet		✓
top		✓
stop	✓	

The rationale behind this approach is to direct the child's attention to the omission of /s/ (raising right hand) as a general pattern of behavior. Later, in the discussion on procedures for teaching production (Chapter 5), there are further suggestions regarding the acquisition of /s/ before stops.

Another child was found to have the following articulatory behavior:

Standard sound	Substitution
/v/	/b/
/f/	/p/
/s/	/t/
/z/	/d/
/ʃ/ correctly used	
/ʒ/ correctly used	
/θ/ correctly used	
/ð/ correctly used	

The above record indicates that this child discriminates and uses correctly four fricatives. Four other fricatives, namely, /v, f, s, z/, are not used correctly. Subsequent testing reveals that each fricative cannot be discriminated from its respective error substitution; i.e., there is no discrimination between the sounds of the respective pairs, /v-b/, /f-p/, /s-t/, and /z-d/. Furthermore, the tests reveal that correct discriminations are made between all combinations of /v, f, s, z/. The child discriminates between /v/ and /f/, /v/ and /s/, /v/ and /z/, /f/ and /s/, and so on.

We conclude that this child can discriminate easily between place of articulation and voice, for stops and fricatives. Note that /v/ is substituted by /b/, not /p/, and /s/ by /t/, not /p/, etc. What the child is unable to discriminate is the difference (contrast) between the stop feature and the fricative feature for the labial and apical places of articulation. This child's discrimination errors do not stem from an inability to discriminate sounds, but rather from an inability to discriminate between the stop-fricative feature contrast, for a number of sounds. The training should reflect this fact.

Initially, the stop-fricative contrast should be taught. There are two parts in the teaching of the stop-fricative contrasts. First, select a single contrast, say /v-b/, and train this difference using the procedures discussed above. Second, teach the cataloguing of the fricatives and the stops as separate sets.

Let us examine the first stage in this procedure, which involves a contrast of a single pair. We might develop the following sequence:

1. /b/   /ʃ/
2. /b/   /f/
3. /b/   /v/

In the second step the stop-fricative contrast is taught across all four pairs. We might develop the following conceptualization training scheme:

Stimulus	Left hand	Right hand
/v/	✓	
/ʃ/	✓	
/θ/	✓	
/f/	✓	
/b/		✓
/p/		✓
/s/	✓	
/z/	✓	
/t/		✓
/d/		✓

If transfer to the other stop-fricative contrasts does not develop, that is, if the child is unable to solve this problem, we would recommend taking two additional steps. First, limit the conceptualization training to the four labials /p, b, f, v/. If transfer to the /p-f/ pair does not take place after a reasonable number of trials, return to the single pair approach for one of the pairs.

The sequence for the /p-f/ contrast might be:

1. /p/   /ʒ/
2. /p/   /v/
3. /p/   /f/

At this point it is worth a try to repeat the conceptualization training.

SOUND DISCRIMINATION PRINCIPLE 9

Whenever articulatory errors follow a pattern, select two sounds that reflect this pattern. Employ discrimination procedures with these two sounds. Subsequent to this training, begin conceptualization training. If conceptualization training fails to produce generalization, select another contrasting pair for discrimination training.

Clinical Example

There is the possibility that, in some instances, discriminations can be made, but for some reason a child has failed to utilize the rule in production. For example, a child might not produce final stops, as instanced below:

Word	Child's response
stop	omit /p/
let	omit /t/
rock	omit /k/
rub	omit /b/
bead	omit /d/
rug	omit /g/

The rule is: Word-final stops are omitted.

Let us assume that we have tested this child's discrimination of word-final stops. We find that he can discriminate capably between words with and without final stops when the final stops are released with slight aspiration. He can hear the difference between "bea" and "beat," "bay" and "bake," and so on. We may conclude that discrimination is not a problem.

When there is no deficiency in discrimination, we should concentrate our energies on conceptualization. A segment of the training sequence might be as follows:

Word	Left hand	Right hand
bay	√	
bake		√
bea	√	
beat		√
knee	√	
need		√

If the child does not add final stops subsequent to intensive conceptualization training, we would recommend production training. Select one sound, for example /t/, and teach this sound in the final position of a large number of words. Acquisition should be fairly rapid because the /t/ is produced correctly as a word initial.

After the /t/ is learned, repeat the conceptualization training, and then, once again, test for generalization of production for the remaining final stops. As discussed in the next chapter, a good degree of generalization should result, with a minimum of emphasis on production.

SOUND DISCRIMINATION PRINCIPLE 10

If it is found that a child's articulatory errors are rule governed and that there is no difficulty in sound discrimination, set up a program of conceptualization training. If conceptualization training is not effective, begin production training with one sound. When this one sound is mastered, try conceptualization training once again.

CHAPTER 5

Teaching the Production of Sounds

Discrimination is an important prerequisite for the achievement of production skills. Under certain conditions discrimination training may lead to changes in production. In other instances "direct" attention must be given to the teaching of articulatory responses.

In Chapter 4 we indicated that the effect of discrimination training should not be underestimated. We called attention to the fact that children learn to articulate because the communicative process demands that they listen well to their mother's speech, and because mothers will not respond appropriately to their child's speech unless it is momentarily intelligible.

An inappropriate response by the mother will lead to further analysis on the part of the child. He will tend to listen more carefully, and he will try to respond more accurately. Good clinical practice should capture this important fact when production is taught.

As a matter of fact, discrimination training cannot be avoided in the "direct" teaching of production. Every time we produce a sound or word, we are providing auditory practice. True, contrasting pairs are not always involved, yet there is continuous bombardment of the auditory sense. There is also every possibility that, as a new sound is learned, it is contrasted with the sounds already in memory. Similarly, phonetic placements methods, positioning of a child's articulator by the clinician, is 90% auditory. It is auditory because the clinician produces the sound before manipulation and during maintenance training, and, as in every method for teaching production, there is auditory feedback from one's own response.

If learning to produce sounds relies so heavily on the auditory component, why do we call it production training? We do so because we emphasize three practices. First, we ask the child to respond, rather than waiting for him to respond. In the words of B. F. Skinner, production training is a *controlled operant*. Second, we are more deliberate with our reinforcements of correct responses. Our social rewards, such as "That's good," or "You may play this game now," are contrived and systematic. The technology of reinforcement we owe, in large part, also to B. F. Skinner (see Skinner, 1938), whose writings often have been misunderstood. Many parents and teachers have told me that reinforcement means popping an "M & M" chocolate into a child's mouth. We will not begin a technical debate on reinforcement theory, except to say that it can be used in very meaningful ways. An elementary school principal, whom I know, permits children to receive points for good work and good behavior. The points are exchanged for reinforcements, a certain number of which allows the student to see the principal and engage him in conversation for a few minutes.

Third, we isolate the stimulus input in a more systematic way than is usually true of discrimination training. We may ask the child, as we shall see below, to exaggerate parts of sounds, non-English sounds or unusual sounds, as steps in learning to produce English sounds. In summary, then, production training is more direct and more concentrated than discrimination training.

We can now explore procedures to facilitate articulatory acquisition. In the first chapter several testing procedures were discussed; these are now to be presented as production principles.

PRODUCTION PRINCIPLE 1

Determine if the child is stimulable. The determination is made by asking him to imitate the clinician's productions of the sound he does not use correctly. If the child can imitate correctly, there is no need to apply the specialized discrimination techniques discussed above. All that seems to be necessary is to demonstrate to the child that he can say the sounds and to indicate when his pronunciations are correct. We recommend that the clinician contrive circumstances in which the child is eager to talk. Then the clinician should respond appropriately to correct productions and inappropriately to incorrect productions.

PRODUCTION PRINCIPLE 2

Some children, to use the phraseology of Milisen, are not immediately stimulable. The next tactic is to search for isolated instances in which the phoneme is said correctly. It is generally recommended that blends and unusual contexts be tested. Not a great deal of time should be spent in this endeavor. One session would seem to be sufficient.

If we are fortunate to find a context or two in which the error sound is correctly produced, generalization procedures, as discussed in the next chapter, are recommended. Sometimes we are not so fortunate, and we need to restrict our search to phonetic features.

Clinical Example

If no single lexical or phonological context can be found in which the error sound is correctly uttered, the search for appropriate phonetic features should begin. Let us assume that a young child omits /s/. The /s/ is composed of the following features: voiceless, apicoalveolar, and fricative. Determine if these features occur in the child's utterances by examining as many sounds as possible. We may find, for example, that these features occur in the following sounds:

Sound	Feature
/t/	voiceless, apicoalveolar
/n/	apicoalveolar
/ʃ/	voiceless, fricative
/f/	voiceless, fricative

For non-organically involved children, the fricative feature that is produced at the palate for /ʃ/, or at the lips for /f/, should be generalizable to the alveolar ridge, as in the production of /s/. Therefore, this child's potential for learning /s/ seems to be great. Generalization procedures would seem to be in order.

Suppose a young child were found to have the following errors:

Sound	Child's response
/tʃ/	/t/
/dʒ/	/d/
/ʃ/	/ʃ/ (correct)
/ʒ/	/ʒ/ (correct)
/t/	/k/
/d/	/g/
/-ts/	/-ts/ (correct)
/-dz/	/-dz/ (correct)

The affricates, /tʃ/ and /dʒ/, are misarticulated, but the four sounds /t, ʃ, d, ʒ/ appear in the child's record. The affricates /-ts/ and /-dz/ also appear. This child would seem to have great potential for learning /tʃ/ and /dʒ/ because the separate components that make up these sounds can be produced. Also, this child can combine stops and fricatives to produce affricates.

PRODUCTION PRINCIPLE 3

If a sound is misarticulated, and also is not correct in any of many contexts tested, search for the appearance of features that make up the correct sound. If the features are present, the potential for learning the correct sound would seem to be great.

At this point it is of interest to reflect on the error itself, a point not often stressed in introductory texts on articulation. It is conceivable that the error may be an important influence on our choice of training procedures.

Clinical Examples

Two children misarticulate /s/, but one child substitutes /θ/ for /s/, and the other substitutes /k/ for /s/. These errors are described below:

Child 1: θ/s

Phonetic features of /θ/	*Phonetic features of /s/*
voiceless	voiceless
apex	apex
dental*	alveolar
fricative	fricative

In the case of the first child, only the dental position, marked with an asterisk above, needs to be altered. As we can see below, the second child's error substitution is substantially different from the /s/:

Child 2: k/s

Phonetic features of /k/	*Phonetic features of /s/*
voiceless	voiceless
dorsum*	apex
velum*	alveolar
stop*	fricative

In the case of the second child, three features, denoted with asterisks, need to be altered. It seems that it would be more difficult to modify the error of the second child than the first child. However, to my knowledge, the effect on learning of phonetic feature disparity, as measured by the difference between the error sound and the standard sound, has never been tested.

In examining this hypothesis it would be important to take into account the presence of other features in the child's repertoire. If the second child possesses sounds containing the phonetic features that define /s/, then he may not differ in learning capability from the first child. Sounds that contain the missing features would include: /n, z, f, v, t, d, ʃ, ʒ/.

It would also be of interest to know whether stimulability is correlated with the number of correct features of the error sound. For example, would the first child respond to stimulation better than the second child?

Until further information is available, we hesitate to present a principle. Nonetheless, the concept regarding the features of the error are relevant for our next topic, which we call *shaping*. Shaping is a psychological procedure that involves changing features. It would seem reasonable to assume that the fewer features that need to be changed, the greater the chances of learning.

There may be instances in which one or two features of the correct sound are absent, and these features, after an exhaustive search, are not found in any contexts. For example, if /s/ is substituted by /θ/, only one feature is missing, and that is alveolar contact. The features voiceless and frication, as well as use of the apex of the tongue, appear in the production of /θ/. A thorough search is made, and none of the sounds, for which alveolar positioning is essential, is present. As you might guess, this child has a severe articulation disorder.

At this point there are many options open to us. We might teach alveolar contact by phonetic placement, either by instruction or direct manipulation. A tongue depressor can be used to press the tongue tip against the alveolar ridge. Additionally, we can describe the location of the alveolar area and ask the child to position his tongue there. Although children can be taught alveolar placement in these two ways, there is no guarantee that these isolated movements will transfer to speech production without extensive practice with speech movements, unlike the procedure described directly below. A third alternative is to begin a series of imitation trials. Again, we do not recommend imitation practice over an extended period of time. There is no point in having a child imitate when it is clear he repeatedly makes the same mistakes. We better try something else.

The procedure we recommend is called *shaping*. We begin with a simple response and gradually move toward the desired response (Winitz, 1969).

Consider again the child who substitutes /θ/ for /s/ and has no alveolar sounds. As shown below the /θ/ is a competitor of /s/. Competition may be minimized by selecting phonetic contexts that are unfamiliar to the child and that do not provoke the /θ/ sound.

In the case of /s/ a simple response that is non-competitive is the inspirated /s/. Have the child imitate a "sucked-in" /s/. We symbolize an inspirated sound with ← and an expirated sound by →. The training program would be:

1. s̰
2. s̰   s̰i
3.   s̰i

In this program, begin with s̰. As soon as the child can make this sound well, move to s̰ s̰i , inspiration and expiration made quickly in succession. Finally, the inspiration is eliminated, symbolized by s̰i .

A child whom I saw several years ago was unable to produce the velar stops, /k/ and /g/. Training began with the inspirated velar fricative, [χ], which sounds like a snore, and within a short period of time /k/ and /g/ could be produced. We can symbolize the training sequence as follows:

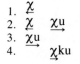

In this case the child is taught a fricative that is a simple and easily produced response. Transfer is made from a velar fricative to a velar stop. With some careful thought, the reader can generate additional programs.

PRODUCTION PRINCIPLE 4

When a feature is not present in the child's repertoire of sounds, select a response that is easily taught and that also contains the missing feature. Gradually, this feature is transferred to the intended sound by making use of the principle of shaping.

Whether we shape phonetic features or not, we should minimize interference from the error sound. In two studies (Winitz and Bellerose, 1965; Leonard, 1973) it was found that children acquire new sounds rapidly when they are taught as nonsense words.

Furthermore, Powell and McReynolds (1969) have found that transfer from nonsense syllables to words can be accomplished easily. That sounds should be learned in syllables before they are learned in words has been advocated for some time (Van Riper, 1939), although the theoretical reason was not clearly stated. It seems that nonsense words do not usually elicit the error sound, perhaps because it is a context in which the error sound has not been learned.

Clinical Example

A young child substitutes /w/ for /r/. The child is provided with attractively colored nonsense objects (see Gerber, 1973, for more detail). They are called nonsense objects because they are unfamiliar items. The child might be shown the following:

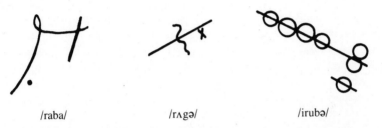

/rabə/   /rʌgə/   /irubə/

The child next learns to pick up the correct object on command. After the object can be identified, the child is asked to imitate the clinician's pronunciation of each object. Eventually, these items are introduced into sentences. I would recommend that at least twenty nonsense items, introduced over several sessions, be learned well in isolation and in sentences before instituting transfer.

Transfer is an easy matter. After the child feels comfortable with these nonsense words in conversation, "strategic" phonemes are deleted. For /rʌgə/ the final /ə/ is deleted by asking the child to say /rʌg/. If the child experiences no difficulty with /r/ at this point, he is next shown a picture of a rug and asked to imitate the clinician's pronunciation of this item. Gradually, additional nonsense words are transformed into words.

PRODUCTION PRINCIPLE 5

Nonsense words reduce interference from the error sound. The use of nonce words will increase the rate at which speech sounds are acquired.

A commonly recognized principle of learning theory is reinforcement. Very simply, a reinforcer is viewed by learning theorists as a contingency that governs the acquisition and repeatability of human behavior.

Material rewards are infrequently employed in public school settings. Often we reinforce correct articulatory responses by permitting a child to play a game or by giving social commendations. A verbal "pat on the back" is probably all that is necessary for young children.

The reinforcement principle can be misused in the practice of articulatory remediation when the behaviors that are to be reinforced are not well spelled out. We have to decide in advance what to regard as an acceptable response. Once we decide, there can be no hedging.

Clinical Example

A young child misarticulates the /s/ sound. Using procedures outlined above, we have taught him to produce an inspirated /s/, symbolized by /s̲/. He is now ready for the next step, /s̲ s̲i̲/. We can only tell the child that he is correct if indeed the /s/ is produced correctly. If we respond by saying, "Almost right," "You almost had it that time," or "Pretty good, make it better next time," we mislead the child. He is unclear as to how he is "almost right" but "not quite right."

It is best to tell the child to listen to each stimulus and to try to match it. If he continues to fail, it may be that the steps in the program are too large. Perhaps they should be redefined, or another program or set of procedures should be employed. To define what we regard as a correct response, and to stick with it, are critically important. If we do this, we will find that our children are more attentive because they are not satisfied until we commend them. Partial commendation (e.g., "That's all right, you almost got it") may satisfy a child to the point that he is not motivated to try to perfect his response.

PRODUCTION PRINCIPLE 6

Reinforcement plays an important role in the teaching of speech sound productions. A child should be informed almost immediately after he produces a sound as to whether or not it is correct. By reinforcing only correct responses, as predetermined by the clinician, the child will strive to achieve perfection and will not be satisfied with less than accurate behavior.

CHAPTER 6

Phonetic Context and Coarticulation

The seminal article of Spriestersbach and Curtis (1951) called attention to the fact that children are not consistent in their errors. An individual child, they report, may produce a sound incorrectly in one context and correctly in another context. Spriestersbach and Curtis found that /s/ and /r/ are often produced correctly in blends, such as /sp/ and /tr/, respectively, even though they are uttered incorrectly in singles, such as in the words soup and rabbit.

It is now a generally recognized fact (see Daniloff and Hammarberg, 1973) that sounds are produced in parallel, what McDonald (1964) referred to as overlapping articulatory movements. Parallel transmission means that the acoustic characteristics of more than one sound will occur in the same time interval. Below, the parallel transmission of two phonemes, denoted here as A and B, are illustrated:

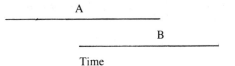

Phonemes A and B intersect during about half of their individual durations. An example of serial transmission is given below:

A _____

                                    B _____

                Time

Rather than sharing the acoustic time continuum, phonemes A and B are in sequence.

Phoneticians have suggested that listeners would be unable to process speech as rapidly as is commonly the case (about 15 to 20 phonemes/ second), if phonemic transmission were not in parallel. Parallel transmission more than doubles the speed at which phonemes can be identified.

In some fairly recent studies, perceptual evidence has been gathered which demonstrates that listeners can detect neighboring phonemes before their production. Ali et al. (1971) found that listeners could easily identify whether or not a nasal consonant followed a vowel when only the vowel was present. These investigators chopped off the final nasal in consonant-vowel sequences, and still the nasality was detectable on the vowel. We would have expected this result only for those speakers who have excessive anticipatory nasality. Winitz, Scheib, and Reeds (1973) found that listeners could identify the following vowel on the aspiration portion of stop consonants. The vowels /i, u, a/ were removed from initial /t, p, k/. The listeners heard only the consonantal portions, and yet identified the vowels fairly well.

COARTICULATION

That neighboring sounds affect each other has been long acknowledged by linguists. A cover term for this phenomenon is *assimilation*. In the disciplines of acoustic and physiological phonetics, the more popular term is *coarticulation*. The reason the term coarticulation is gaining favor is because it implies a basic physiological (articulatory) process whereas assimilation is a term more aptly used to describe phonetic alterations. Coarticulation refers directly to the role of the speech motor process. What is observed is the apparent influence of phonetic segments on neighboring phonetic segments. The segments are not produced independently, but observed to be coarticulated.

Rules can be used to describe phonetic variations. The nasalization of vowels preceding nasals (e.g., /m, n, ŋ/) is regarded as an instance of assimilation. Sometimes alveolar stops are eliminated following nasal sounds. The phonological rule that expresses these two facts is: Vowels before nasals are nasalized, and nasals are eliminated when preceding alveolar stops (i.e., /d/ and /t/). An example of a deleted alveolar is the segment /kæt/ often substituted for "can't" in running speech. Coarticulation refers to the physiological process of assimilative nasality. It describes the mechanics of phonetic production as well as the speech motor code that governs articulation.

Described here are two types of coarticulation. The first is *left to right* coarticulation, schematized as A B. The symbol A B means that the utterance of phoneme A affects the pronunciation of phoneme B. The following are examples of left to right coarticulation in English:

1. The /j/ in *you* becomes /ʃ/ when it follows /t/, as in *won't you*.
2. The /r/ in *train* is realized as voiceless, following the (voiceless) /t/.
3. The /t/ in *bathtub* is dentalized because it follows a /θ/.
4. The /f/ in *campfire* is often a bilabial fricative because it follows the (bilabial) /p/.
5. The /p/ in *spoon* is unaspirated because it follows /s/.

A second type of coarticulation is a *right to left* adjustment, symbolized as A B. The notation A B implies that phoneme B, which has not yet been uttered, will affect the pronunciation of phoneme A. The following are examples of right to left coarticulation:

1. A vowel before a nasal consonant is often nasalized.
2. A /t/ before a back vowel, as in *two,* is rounded; before a front vowel it is not rounded.
3. A /k/ before /i/ is made more forward than a /k/ before /u/.
4. A vowel preceding a voiced stop is usually longer than a vowel preceding a voiceless stop.
5. The /l/ in *William* is forward because it precedes /j/.

There are at least two processes (Curtis, 1970) that may account for the observed behavior we call coarticulation: a) physiological constraints stemming from structural inertia and anatomical restrictions, and b) a complex preprogramming mechanism.

Inertia, a term used in classical mechanics, refers to the persistence of objects in rest or in motion. The first law of Newtonian mechanics states that bodies remain at rest or in motion unless an external force is applied. An instance of physiological inertia in speech involves the /it-ik/ contrast. The tongue is high and forward for the production of /i/, then continues its forward movement for the production of /t/. To produce /k/ the tongue must reverse its direction before the dorsum of the tongue can make contact with the velum. For this reason, the contact for /i/ preceding /t/ may be different than for /i/ preceding /k/. Furthermore, the effect of the following stop, in this case /t/ or /k/, is a right to left constraint, which, for rapid rates of speech, intensifies the phonetic variations of /i/. Evidence provided by Kent and Moll (1972) suggests that, for at least one of the two speakers they studied, a rapid rate of speech produced undershooting of the maximum alveolar placement of /z/ in the contexts /izi/, /uzu/, and /aza/. In general, the undershooting was greatest for the /u/ and /a/ vowels. There is also considerable acoustic data showing the effect of phonetic context. In one investigation (Stevens, House, and Paul, 1966) consonantal environment affected the acoustic values of vowels (formants), which, according to the investigations, reflected mechanoinertial factors.

Anatomical restriction refers to the fact that there are certain speech productions that are impossible because the articulators cannot produce simultaneous activities. The lips, for example, cannot be rounded and retracted at the same time. Also it is difficult to round a low central vowel, such as /a/, because the mandible is depressed. Kent and Moll (1972) observed that, for /d/ and /z/, the tongue body constrains tongue tip movement. In conclusion, "phonetic context" is simply a frame of reference; varying articulatory configurations are constrained by physiological inertia and anatomical restrictions.

The term coarticulation has come to be identified with the complexity of the articulation programming process. At this point, explanations with some degree of consistency are absent (see Daniloff and Hammarberg, 1973); however, there are a great number of interesting observations.

Lip Rounding and Nasals

Daniloff and Moll (1968) tracked the production of lip rounding by carefully analyzing x-ray motion pictures of a series of words and phrases that terminated with the /u/ vowel. They found that the incipience of lip rounding for /u/ began several phonemes in advance of its production. Below, we list several of the phonetic strings studied by Daniloff and Moll. An arrow below the phoneme indicates the point at which the lips began to round:

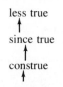

less true

since true

construe

Two interesting conclusions were drawn by Daniloff and Moll. First, coarticulation of lip rounding can extend over as many as four phonemes; and second, the presence of word and syllable boundaries did not affect the initiation of lip rounding movements.

In a later investigation Kent, Carney, and Severeid (1974) made an interesting observation regarding the articulatory gestures of nasals. From cinefluorographic films they charted the timing of velar movements relative to the oral constriction of the nasal, and the neighboring vowels and consonants.

Generally, Kent and his colleagues found that, as lingual contact is being made for the nasal consonant, the velum is returning from its lowered position. For example, the sequence of articulatory productions for the noun contract is as follows:

1. The velum begins to lower with the release of /k/.
2. As the tongue is positioned for /a/, the velum lowering is complete.
3. Velar elevation and tongue tip movement for /n/ occur at about the same time.

The dynamics of articulatory production for lip rounding of back vowels and velar-oral timing in vowel-nasal-consonant sequences evidence a similarity. In both instances, articulatory gestures for lip rounding and nasality are in advance of what generally would be regarded as the central tendency value for these sounds. However, there are differences, which Kent, Carney, and Severeid (1974) specify well. Early initiation of velar raising must occur, or there will be a delay in the production of the following consonant, especially for sequences such as /nt/. Build-up in intraoral pressure cannot begin until there is near velopharyngeal closure. A delay in the development of pressure would result in a delay in the production of the oral consonant. In this instance, then, constraints of time account for the anticipatory behavior.

It is interesting to note that Netsell and Daniel's (1974) research and their review of the literature on reaction time suggest that at least 125 to 200 milliseconds is necessary to initiate a speech production. Their findings suggest that time constraints, independent of a particular articulatory act, are responsible for a certain degree of the anticipatory behavior observed in right to left coarticulation.

Underlying Mechanisms of Speech Movements

The above descriptions of articulatory movements unquestionably recommend a complex motor control system, which organizes in a cohesive and hierarchical fashion the commands issued to the speech structures. Speech production can be viewed as the terminal phase of the language act, a process initiated by an idea, molded into a syntax, and finally converted into neuromotor units. A variety of models (e.g., Kozhevnikov and Chistovich, 1965; Henke, 1967; Liberman et al., 1967; Wickelgren, 1969) has been proposed to account for the dynamics of articulatory encoding. We can regard these models as hypotheses about the underlying mechanisms that govern speech movements, the output of which, phoneticians try to capture in their precise transcriptions.

An interpretation of the last few phases of this process is as follows:

Stage	Level of Encoding	Description	Example
1	Terminal syntactic level	Sentence unit	"Worthy phoneticians experiment"
2	Abstract phonological level	Distinctive features assigned by rule given a base form	w⟶ $\begin{bmatrix} +\text{ labial} \\ +\text{ voice} \\ \vdots \end{bmatrix}$
3	Abstract phonetic level	Speaker-hearer's interpretation of an utterance	In features: $\begin{bmatrix} \text{`` } +\text{ labial} & -\text{ voice} \\ +\text{ voice} & \ldots+\text{ apical} \\ +\text{ semivowel} & +\text{ alveolar} \\ & +\text{ stop} \end{bmatrix}$ In phonetics: "/w ...t/"
4	Neuromotor commands	Actualization of target phonetic values reflecting coarticulation and timing properties	"The /r/ in 'worthy' is produced in the dental region; it reflects right to left coarticulation, symbolized as /ɝ ð/"
5	Production	Acoustic and physiological record	"Spectrograph-oscillograph-cineradiograph"

The above schema should be regarded only as tentative. First, we have not specified the length of the string over which each of the hypothesized cognitive and physiological processes are presumed to occur. For example, at stage 4, is the coarticulated string a phrase, morpheme, syllable, word, or as yet some unidentifiable unit? Second, considerable mixing of the levels probably occurs as speech is being produced. It would be naive to regard stages 1 through 5 as operating in a strictly linear fashion. Third, this model does not permit a clear distinction between the motor component, the hierarchical physiological organization of phonetic strings, and the phonological level, the abstract rules that govern phonetic strings. Undoubtedly, there are phonological rules that result from inherent restrictions on the speech apparatus, and there are coarticulation behaviors that reflect the phonological rules of an individual language.

Of immediate concern to us is the restriction placed on features that are contiguous or nearly contiguous. Consider the string of phonemes in the phrases "a bit" and "a kit." In "a bit" forward movement of /i/ begins to occur as the /b/ begins to be formed. In "a kit" the lingual backing necessary for /k/ delays any forward movement of the anterior portion of the tongue.

In one investigation of competing articulatory movements, Daniloff and Moll (1968) found that lip rounding for /u/ in "a plume" provided somewhat of a mystery. Lip rounding began in two spots, on the /l/, and as the tongue moved to the /u/, symbolized as:

$$/plum/$$

Daniloff and Moll suggest that there are two protrusion gestures (their metric for lip rounding) for this word. As to why the lips returned to a neutral position between the completion of /l/ and the start of /u/ is not clear, but there may be two reasons. First, it is possible that the initial gesture of lip protusion was for /p/. In that case /l/ was achieved before a change in labial placement could be made, an example of left to right coarticulation. Second, in some contexts initial /l/ phones, as pronounced in English, may require, as Daniloff and Moll suggested, a certain degree of lip protrusion. As an example, the investigators observed lip rounding for the /l/ in "less true."

We have discussed in considerable detail the bimodal occurrence of lip protrusion in "a plume" because it brings us to an important point. When there is a conflict between two or more articulatory features, articulatory commands are executed in sequence. Anticipatory left to right coarticulation does not occur for a particular feature if a contradictory feature intervenes. An obvious example involves the contrast between "renew" and "read new." In "renew" anticipation of /n/ produces assimilated nasality for the first vowel, /i/, whereas in "read new" nasality does not occur for /i/ because /d/, an oral sound, intervenes. The amount of nasality, generated by left to right coarticulation, should be the same for the second vowel of the two words. In summary, then, coarticulation is maximized when competing commands are absent.

PHONETIC CONTEXT PRINCIPLE 1

Coarticulation can be maximized in the teaching of new articulatory movements by taking cognizance of conflicting articulatory gestures.

The principle of coarticulation, as stated above, does not distinguish between right to left (R-L) and left to right (L-R) coarticulation. The discussion so far has singled out R-L coarticulation with the clear implication that L-R coarticulation produces less than satisfactory results.

As a matter of fact, an acquisition experiment in which a comparison between R-L and L-R coarticulation for comparable speech sounds and environments has never been conducted. However, L-R and R-L environments, using standard testing procedures, were examined by Zehel et al. (1972). They observed that R-L coarticulated contexts produce a larger number of correct /s/ productions than L-R coarticulated contexts. This finding was especially true when the adjacent sound was alveolar. The reason, we conjecture, is because R-L coarticulation is primarily an anticipatory process whereas L-R coarticulation reflects the compatibility between two adjacent phonemes. An example of compatibility is the sequence /θt/ in the word bathtub (phonetically /bæθt̪əb/). The sequence /θt/ comprises a cohesive unit, which no doubt is encoded at a fairly high level (stage 3, phonological level, or stage 4, coarticulation level). Let us assume it is encoded at stage 4 as a phonetic rule: Whenever /t/ follows /θ/ it is dentalized. Then at stage 5, this rule would be realized as part of the overall articulatory plan.

As is clearly obvious, the apical contacts for /θ/ and /t/ cannot be made simultaneously although the physiological position for the body of the tongue is probably the same. Therefore, the phonetic features that are in conflict involve the articulations of the apicoalveolar and apicodental contacts. Alveolar positioning, of course, could be made following /θ/, and probably does for some individuals. The fact that the contact for /t/ is dental, rather than alveolar, suggests advanced planning. Advanced planning, then, is not synonymous with anticipatory movements. Planning takes place with both R-L and L-R coarticulation.

Clinical Example

In order to explain how anticipatory movements are essential in training, let us consider a child with /r/ errors. A phonetic context that maximizes the forward positioning of /r/ is /irdʌgə/. The child in question substitutes /w/ for /r/. When asked to imitate /r/ the child utters /w/ except for contexts similar to /irdʌgə/. We note that in these contexts the /w/ substitution is eliminated after several trials. What seems to be happening here? Apparently, movements relevant to the production of /r/ are generated in advance of /d/, that is, where /w/ would normally occur, because /d/ follows /r/. The features of apicoalveolar and voiced would be regarded as relevant ones. Note, however, that there is no reason to assume that the /rd/ context will foster retroflexion. Yet the fact that alveolar movements are anticipated increases the likelihood that retroflexion will be imitated. In contrast /irgʌdə/ minimizes front sound positioning, since the anticipation of /g/

pulls back the body of the tongue after /i/ is produced. Thus, for the interval between /i/ and /g/, that is, /i. . .g/, gestures that are in conflict with /w/ are not present.

Conceivably, L-R coarticulation, which does not involve anticipatory gestures, may facilitate articulatory acquisition. Above, we suggested that /irdʌgə/ is a phonetic constellation in which R-L coarticulation facilitates the acquisition of /r/. If we reverse /d/ and /r/ to form /idrʌgə/, the /r/ now follows the /d/. Because /d/ precedes /r/ any effect /d/ has on /r/ is an aftertrace: There normally is no break (return to a neutral position) in the apicoalveolar positioning of /d/ as /r/ is being formed. However, there is no guarantee that a smooth L-R transition, such as when /d/ follows /r/, will facilitate the production of /r/. Also, it is unlikely that anticipation of /w/ will be nullified by L-R constraints.

We may tentatively conclude that R-L coarticulation facilitates acquisition more effectively than L-R coarticulation, although there is only the tangential evidence of Zehel et al. (1972) to support this belief.

In addition to facilitating acquisition, R-L coarticulation may improve generalization. As indicated above, L-R coarticulation is largely a function of mechanical and inertial constraints. R-L coarticulation reflects less these constraints of classical mechanics, and, therefore, greater control over articulatory patterns might be expected. Thus, it would seem that generalization across phonetic contexts would be swifter for R-L coarticulation than for L-R coarticulation.

PHONETIC CONTEXT PRINCIPLE 2

At this time, the evidence seems to suggest that articulatory change can be best affected when one or more features of the correct sound are anticipated. Anticipation probably facilitates articulation change because the anticipated features are retained in the phonetic slot of the error sound. For this reason, R-L contexts are to be preferred to L-R contexts in the modification of articulatory behavior.

This issue was thoroughly discussed in a thoughtful exchange between McNutt and Keenan (1970) and Shriner and Daniloff (1971). The argument stemmed from a remark by Shriner, Holloway, and Daniloff (1969) that was incidently attached to the discussion section of a paper on language and articulation.

Shriner and Daniloff, using coarticulation as a frame of reference, commented that the /n/ phoneme in the phrase one red ball (/wʌn rɛd bɔl/) will facilitate production of the /r/ in the word red. McNutt and Keenan

(1970) acknowledged that the cohesive aspects of coarticulation should be put to good use, but neither Shriner and Daniloff, nor McNutt and Keenan, recommended R-L coarticulation. In fact, Shriner and Daniloff preferred L-R coarticulation as evidenced by their statement (Shriner and Daniloff, 1971, p. 442):

> . . . the /n/ is being used to facilitate production of the error in question, which in this case is /r/. The /n/ should precede or be immediately adjacent to the error in question, preferably preceding than following.

Later in their rebuttal, Shriner and Daniloff (1971) acknowledged that the vowel following /r/ can act as a facilitator. Yet they clearly emphasized L-R over R-L coarticulation. In our discussion above, we indicated that R-L coarticulation is preferred.

One point, offered by McNutt and Keenan, should be explored further. They recommended avoiding the use of /w/ before /r/ because /w/ is a common error for /r/. Possibly, they said, the /w/ may persist, that is, move forward in the string, thus obstructing the formation of /r/. Shriner and Daniloff countered that the coarticulatory effects of /w/ on "one" would be minimal; that is, it would not extend beyond the nasal. Because we have no data on coarticulatory effects of strings like this one for /r/-defective populations, there is no way to settle this issue. I would tend to side with McNutt and Keenan, but for a different reason: The /w/ may transfer by its very presence to the slot of the correct sound. Thus, for psychological reasons, we offer the third principle of phonetic context.

PHONETIC CONTEXT PRINCIPLE 3

Avoid selecting phrases or sentences in which a sound similar to the error substitution is adjacent to or near the position occupied by the error sound.

Admittedly, our rationale has a psychological rather than a physiological basis. As we saw in the preceding chapter, the error response must be inhibited in the early phases of training. That is why we suggest using nonce words. Elicitation of the error would seem to work only at cross purposes.

CHAPTER 7

Transfer from One Context to the Next

After a child acquires a new sound, his next step is a very difficult one. He must learn to transfer his correct production to a number of new contexts. Initially the new contexts involve phonetic environments. Later they include words, sentences, and conversational speech both inside and outside the clinic. These contexts often define the order of training in traditional speech pathology programs (Wing and Heimgartner, 1973).

In Chapter 5 we altered this sequence by recommending that nonce items be mastered in conversational speech before a new sound is introduced into words. At this point let us retrace our steps and examine the contexts in which articulatory responses are learned. Later in this chapter we examine transfer of phonetic features among sounds, and still later, in Chapter 8, we examine the maintenance and recall of sounds.

In the argot of most speech pathology texts, "sounds are learned in isolation and then in syllables." It is unfortunate that this distinction has become codified. The term isolation is false on phonetic grounds. It applies only to continuants. Sounds like the English /p, w, t/ cannot be maintained as isolated segments.

Is there any advantage to teaching continuants as isolated elements? We take the position that sound training in isolation is deleterious to both acquisition and transfer. Thus far, we have developed the position that the acquisition of sounds can be facilitated by the proper phonetic environment. These environments consist of one or perhaps two syllables. It seems, therefore, that syllables have a distinct advantage in articulatory training.

A study by McReynolds (1972) is pertinent to our discussion. Children with /s/ errors were trained with the following sequence: /s/, /sa/, /as/, and /asa/. The training of these four segments was sequential; that is, the training began with /s/ and was followed by /sa/, then /as/, and then /asa/. Each of these four syllables was associated with a nonsense figure. A list of twelve words, four for each word position, was used to test for transfer.[1] The McReynolds paradigm is schematized below:

Train /s/ ↓	*Train /sa/* ↓	*Train /as/* ↓	*Train /asa/* ↓
transfer test	transfer test	transfer test	transfer test
(12 words)	(12 words)	(12 words)	(12 words)

No transfer was observed following /s/ training, even though the children were articulating /s/ correctly more than 90% of the time. On the transfer test following /sa/, the /s/ was produced correctly in a little over one-half of the words. McReynolds does not report to which position transfer was most successful. It is not known, therefore, if transfer to the initial word position was greater than to the medial and final word positions. Furthermore, we do not know whether the initial position is strategically important for initial transfer. Perhaps the rate of transfer would have increased if /as/ (final position) rather than /sa/ (initial position) had followed /s/. Finally, we do not know whether /sa/ would have been acquired easily if it were not preceded by /s/. As indicated earlier (Chapter 6), errors of /s/ are frequently produced correctly in syllabic and blend contexts. This finding suggests that learning a sound in isolation is not critical for learning a sound in syllabic contexts.

In an earlier study, Powell and McReynolds (1969) reported transfer of /s/ from isolation to words, but this finding was largely restricted to one subject. Therefore, we may conclude from the study by McReynolds (1972) that training in isolation is not to be recommended because there is little transfer to words or syllables. In our discussion on phonetic context, we also questioned the wisdom of training in isolation because coarticulatory facilitation is absent.

At this point, it may be instructive to review the reasons why teaching a sound in isolation is no longer recommended. It again should be pointed out that only the continuant sounds can be taught in isolation. Stops and glides can be taught only in syllables.

---

[1]The same twelve words were used throughout the training program—a possible source of error.

Considering the continuant sounds, as well as other sound groups, there are at least three reasons for discouraging the practice of teaching a sound in isolation. First, the facilitating effects of coarticulation cannot be realized. Second, transfer to syllables and words is relatively poor. Third, shaping principles cannot be developed because a variety of contexts is required to make use of this principle. Returning now to the procedures of McReynolds (1972), we can speculate as to why transfer was facilitated. The reasons are: a) /sa/ was learned as a nonsense item, which, as we know, reduces interference from the error sound, and b) /sa/ is a syllable, and rapid transfer to additional syllabic contexts, whether in a word or nonce item, is to be expected.

TRANSFER PRINCIPLE 1

A sound may be acquired in isolation in syllables or nonce words. However, transfer to English words is greatly facilitated if the original training involves syllabic or nonce word contexts.

The fact that we do not advise clinicians to use the principle of isolation in articulatory training in no way violates the *shaping* principle presented in Chapter 5. Even "small" bits of speech should be embedded in contexts that enhance anticipatory movements. When we described the teaching of /s/ we recommended the sequence /s̪/, /s̪ s̪i /, and /s̪i/. It is difficult to teach inspirated vowels, but on expiration the front vowel /i/ was attached in order to facilitate anticipatory gestures common to /s/. The third unit in the /s/ sequence is /si/, the standard beginning point for /s/ training in syllables. Here we regard the employment of /i/ to be important.

In many instances we do not teach small speech segments. Large units are used. For example, the two syllable sequence /is + ti/ might be more useful than the inspirated sequence outlined above. If the /s/ is acquired in /isti/, teaching transfer to blend and non-blend units (e.g., the words step and soap) becomes an important clinical routine.

TRANSFER PRINCIPLE 2

When a sound is acquired in a limited context, it can be transferred to other contexts by varying syllable divisions. Emphasis on syllable divisions has no empirical validity, and it may very well be that transfer will take place after there has been sufficient learning without prescribed syllable training. Only through further research can this issue be decided.

One important consideration in transfer is phonetic similarity. In an early investigation, Winitz and Bellerose (1963, reported in Winitz, 1969) found that children with articulatory errors generalized less when the transfer sounds contained features that they misarticulated. Children with /ʃ/ errors had more difficulty learning the non-English cluster /ʃm/ than children without articulation errors or children who missed *only* the /r/ sound. In one investigation, Elbert, Shelton, and Arndt (1967) taught children to articulate /s/ correctly; they measured, at varying intervals, changes in the performance of /z/ and /r/. Syllables, words, and sentences were included in the transfer tests. Correct responses for /z/ occurred almost from the very beginning and seemed to mirror the production of /s/ throughout training. There was no improvement in the /r/ sound.

In another investigation (Shelton, Elbert, and Arndt, 1967) children with /r/, /s/, and /ʃ/ errors were included. This time instruction was on the /r/ sound. Improvement in /s/ and /ʃ/ was not observed. We may conclude from these three studies that transfer is restricted to phonetically similar items.

It is interesting to note that in two well documented studies (Cairns and Williams, 1972; Singh and Frank, 1972) individual substitution errors of young children evidenced a high degree of phonetic similarity to the respective target sound. Phonetically similar errors are also observed in the speech of young children, as was reported earlier by the parental investigators Smith (1973) and Bullowa (Bullowa, Jones, and Duckert, 1964). Apparently, phonetic similarity governs speech sound development and exerts an important influence on generalization training.

TRANSFER PRINCIPLE 3

Other things being equal, transfer will be directly related to the degree of phonetic similarity between the training sound and the sounds tested for transfer.

Clinical Example

A young child, who substitutes stops for fricatives, is trained to articulate /s/ correctly in words. Subsequent to training, each fricative is again tested to determine if any transfer effects took place:

Standard sound	Error	After training
/s/	/t/	/s/
/z/	/d/	/z/

/ʃ/	/k/	/s/
/ʒ/	/g/	/z/
/f/	/p/	[hw]
/v/	/b/	[hw]
/θ/	omission	[hw]
/ð/	omission	[hw]

For three of the sounds, /z, ʃ, ʒ/, a stop feature was replaced by a fricative feature. Transfer to /z/ was perfect, and, therefore, no further training is needed with this sound. For /ʃ, ʒ/, additional placement training is necessary; /s/ must be changed into /ʃ/, and /ʒ/ into /z/. As can also be observed, /f, v, θ, ð/ require additional placement training.

If, in fact, transfer is as effective as indicated in the above illustration, then it is a phenomenon on which we should capitalize. There is strong evidence from an investigation by McReynolds and Bennett (1972) confirming the reality of feature transfer. Their findings are summarized as follows:

Subject 1		Subject 2		Subject 3	
Train	Transfer of fricative feature	Train	Transfer of voice feature	Train	Transfer of fricative feature
/f/	/v/	/b/	/d/	/ʃ/	/s/
	/s/		/g/		/z/
	/z/				/f/
	/tʃ/				/v/

Transfer was probed by McReynolds and Bennett after the training sound (/f/, /b/, or /ʃ/, as indicated above) was produced correctly 90% of the time. It is important to note that McReynolds and Bennett reported the transfer of features, not sounds. Thus, for subject 1 there was transfer of frication for /v, s, z, tʃ/. This does not mean, however, that these four sounds were produced correctly, only that when they were tested a fricative feature was produced.

TRANSFER PRINCIPLE 4

After the acquisition of a single sound, one or more of its features may transfer to untrained sounds. When this happens, acquisition is facilitated because only the remaining features need to be taught.

Now let us return to the example given above regarding initial /s/ blend errors. Based on the principle of phonetic similarity, I would recommend that, after the mastery of /st/, the order for teaching should be: /sn/, /sl/, /sp/, and /sk/. Before teaching the production of each blend, it is important to check all blends to determine if there has been generalization. For example, if, after teaching /st/, the /sk/ and /sp/ clusters are produced correctly, we should spend some time on these two clusters. This point is emphasized later.

Clinical Example

A young child misarticulates /s/ in initial, medial, and final syllable positions. Which position should be taught first, which second, and which third? The answer to this question really has been given above. Essentially, we have suggested that syllable position is of secondary importance. Rather, selection is guided by syllabic and phonetic contexts. Those coarticulatory contexts that facilitate sound acquisition are to be selected initially. For some allophonic variations, syllable position may be important, but this issue has not yet been settled with regard to generalization learning.

A second question pertains to word position. After an individual sound is learned in syllables and non-word units, the next step is to transfer this sound to words. Again, we can ask which position should be taught first, which second, and which third. This time position refers to word position.

Traditionally, we begin our teaching with the initial word position. This point of view was challenged by Powell and McReynolds (1969). Unfortunately, their investigation provided only preliminary information on this issue. Before examining their approach, we should first establish the transfer paradigms for studying syllable and word position.

The ideal experimental paradigm is summarized as follows:

		Summary of transfer paradigms	
Group	Learn	Transfer 1	Transfer 2
1	Initial position	Medial position	Final position
2	Initial position	Final position	Medial position
3	Medial position	Initial position	Final position
4	Medial position	Final position	Initial position
5	Final position	Medial position	Initial position
6	Final position	Initial position	Medial position

Making use of the above paradigms, we can compare both *success* in transfer and *efficiency* in transfer. Successful transfer is derived by examining the rate at which a sound is acquired in the transfer context. For example, we might compare the rate of transfer—the number of trials required to master a sound—for the medial and final position subsequent to acquisition in the initial position. This comparison pertains to the first two rows and columns above. Here we see that medial and final positions are subsequent to the initial position.

Consider the first and second rows of column 4, in which final position training follows either medial or initial position training. Acquisition in final position can be studied relative to the order in which the initial and medial positions are learned. It is now clear that a great number of comparisons can be made from which the success of transfer can be calculated.

Efficiency of transfer refers to the rate at which a sound is acquired in all three positions regardless of the success rate of transfer. In some cases these two indices may be the same, but, of course, this is an empirical matter. If we compare transfer for groups 2 and 4 (column 3) in our summary of transfer paradigms, it is very possible that the success rate for transfer to the final position is the same when the original learning is the initial or medial positions. If, however, the original learning for the initial position takes much longer than for the medial position, then the total number of trials required for transfer would be less for group 4, for which the original learning was for the medial position and transfer was for the final position.

With this background in mind, we can now return to the Powell and McReynolds (1969) findings. The subjects in this study were first trained to produce /s/ correctly in isolation. Subsequent to syllable training, generalization was tested by comparing correct production of /s/ in words in which /s/ appeared in the initial, medial, and final positions. Transfer to the medial and final positions was equivalent to transfer to the initial position.

The Powell and McReynolds investigation was incomplete as transfer studies go. We can tentatively conclude, however, that, after a sound is mastered in the initial syllable position, there will be equivalent transfer to all three word positions. Regard this last statement as tentative, because phonetic context and allophonic variation may alter the rate of position transfer.

TRANSFER PRINCIPLE 5

After a sound is acquired in the initial syllable position, the rate of successful transfer to the initial, medial, and final positions of words is nearly equivalent. At this point, we would only recommend that teaching begin with the initial syllable position if subsequent research were to show that original learning is most efficient for this position. Needless to say, considerably more research is needed before any definitive statements can be made.

Leonard (1973) investigated a somewhat different topic. He wished to determine whether acquisition of /s/ in English words would be acquired more rapidly if the referent were originally non-English, in contrast to training that involved only English words. Using a nonsense figure as the referent, Leonard trained subjects to acquire /s/ in the segment /saɪn/. Compared to a control group, in which the English word sign was identified to the children by using an appropriate picture, the nonsense referent provided faster learning of /s/. Nonsense referents reduce the possibility that an error sound will be elicited, a conclusion supported by Winitz and Bellerose (1965), as discussed in Chapter 5.

The question of rate of transfer was then examined. Leonard found that more training trials were required to transfer /s/ from non-English referents to English words than were required to teach /s/ in English words from the very beginning. To make this point clear, let us outline two of Leonard's groups as follows:

A: Learn /s/ in /saɪn/ using a nonsense referent; then learn /s/ with "sign" as a referent.

B: Learn /s/ in "sign" as a referent.

The claim that Leonard made was that, although /s/ is acquired faster in the nonsense referent (group A), acquisition in the word "sign" was slower in group A than in group B. A careful examination of the data leads to the opposite conclusion: Nonsense syllable training facilitates the acquisition of the /s/ sound in words. Leonard's erroneous conclusion is based on the results obtained for the transfer stage, the number of trials it took for children in both groups to learn /s/ in the word "sign." In the transfer stage each child had to listen and repeat a story that contained numerous instances of the word "sign." This terminal phase took slightly longer for subjects in group A than for those in group B. However, when the total training program was considered, subjects in group B (the word group) took many more trials to learn to say /s/ correctly than subjects in group A (the nonsense referent group), making invalid the conclusion by Leonard.

TRANSFER PRINCIPLE 6
_____

Transfer to English words is more rapid when the sound is first learned as a nonsense item.

In summary, there are two ways to teach sounds so that interference from the error sound is reduced. Let us schematize the procedure:

	Learn first	*Learn second*
A	Syllable (non-referential)	English word
B	Nonce word	English word

In A, the /s/ sound is first learned in a non-referential syllable, as in /sɪ/, which, of course, has no referent. Then, transfer to English words, such as /sɪt/, is taught. In B, /s/ is taught in the segment /sɪt/, but with a non-English (made up) referent, such as /ɪtsɪt/. Transfer is then to "sit," perhaps using the sequence: /ɪtsɪt/, /tsɪt/, /sɪt/.

I see the two paradigms, A and B, as essentially the same. However, there may be an advantage to using nonce words. Nonce words can be designed so that English words or segments of English words are embedded within the nonce word, as described above and in Chapter 5. A second example is the word seem. Interference is minimized when the unit for the word seem is a simple syllable (/sib/), a non-referential English word (/sim/), or a non-referential unit (/i+sima/). In the last case, phonetic context facilitates acquisition, and transfer simply involves the deletion of initial /i/ and the final /a/ to form the word seem.

Now that the technology of articulatory transfer has been discussed in detail, our next topic pertains to the time at which transfer is implemented.

Clinical Example

A young child has the following substitutions:

Standard sound	Substitution
/s/	/θ/
/z/	/ð/
/t/	/k/
/d/	/g/

Let us assume that the child is taught the /s/ sound and that transfer to /z/, /t/, and /d/ is tested when /s/ is correctly uttered 25% of the time, again at 50%, again at 75%, and finally when no errors occur, or at 100%. Our test protocol appears below:

Percentage of correct /s/ utterances	Percentage of transfer
25%	/z/____/t/____/d/____
50%	/z/____/t/____/d/____
75%	/z/____/z/____/d/____
100%	/z/____/t/____/d/____

The critical question, which faces us now, is when to begin training on /z/, /t/, and /d/. The answer cannot be given easily, especially since the relevant data are unavailable. Let us assume that the following percentages were obtained:

Percentage of correct /s/ utterances	Percentage of transfer
25%	/z/ 10% /t/ 0% /d/ 0%

Percentage of correct	
/s/ utterances	*Percentage of transfer*
50%	/z/ 20% /t/ 0% /d/ 0%
75%	/z/ 40% /t/ 5% /d/ 0%
100%	/z/ 50% /t/ 15% /d/ 10%

Note that /z/ is correctly uttered 50% of the time when /s/ is produced without error, that is, when /s/ is correct 100% of the time. It is possible, of course, that had training on /z/ been implemented at the 25% criterion, progress in /z/ would have closely followed the acquisition of /s/. Again, we do not know because experiments directed to this question have not been conducted.

However, it would seem logical to assume that /z/, and perhaps /t/ and /d/, would be acquired most rapidly if training began before the 100% acquisition point for /s/. The reason is that there are general rules that govern the sound substitutions of /s/, /z/, /t/, and /d/. The rule governing the s/z substitutions is: The apicoalveolar feature becomes apicodental. The rule governing the k/t and d/g substitutions is: The apicoalveolar feature becomes dorsovelar. Two rules, then, can be used to describe the substitution of all four sounds.

Can one rule be used to describe the substitution of all four sounds? It can, but it is much more complex. The one rule might be: The apicoalveolar feature becomes apicodental in the context of a fricative, and dorsovelar in the context of a stop. Let us diagram this rule:

$$\begin{bmatrix} \text{apicoalveolar} \\ \text{fricative} \end{bmatrix} \quad \text{becomes} \quad [\text{apicodental}]$$

$$\begin{bmatrix} \text{apicoalveolar} \\ \text{stop} \end{bmatrix} \quad \text{becomes} \quad [\text{dorsovelar}] \quad (1)$$

The change, then, in the apicoalveolar feature depends on a second feature, which accompanies it in the standard sound. In the case of /s/ and /z/, the fricative feature determines the dental position, and in the case of /t/ and /d/, the stop feature determines the dorsovelar position. That the generalization, albeit minimal occurred for /t/ and /d/, suggests that the two parts of this rule are related. We might express the relations by a second rule:

$$\begin{bmatrix} \text{apicoalveolar} \\ \alpha \text{ continuant} \end{bmatrix} \quad \text{becomes} \quad [\alpha \text{ front}] \quad (2)$$

In the above rule, α can be either positive or negative, that is, +continuant, +front or −continuant, −front. If the apicoalveolar sound is a continuant, /s/ or /z/, the change involves a front sound, /θ/ or /ð/. If the apicoalveolar sound is not a continuant, /t/ or /d/, the change involves a back sound, /k/ or /g/.

In the linguistic sense, rule 2 is the same as rule 1; rule 2 is simply a condensation of rule 1. In the psychological sense, rule 2 may be very different from rule 1. It implies that the frication and stop features are on opposite poles of the same continuum and that the velar and alveolar placements are adequately represented by a front-back contrast. Our transfer tests suggest fairly strongly that linguistic rule 2 is not identical to an underlying psychological process, otherwise changes for /t/ would mirror changes for /z/. Nevertheless, there is some degree of relationship between the errors for /s/ and /z/, and /t/ and /k/, since some change was observed for /t/ and /k/ when attention was only given to /s/. For this reason, we would conclude that training in /t/ and /d/ also should begin before complete mastery of /s/.

CONCLUSIONS

We have, of course, not adequately answered the critical questions, posed above, pertaining to transfer of training and time at which direct intervention should take place. At the present time, all that can be suggested is that, as one or two sounds are taught, transfer to additional sounds should be tested. Psychologists call this *probing for transfer*. If the probes reveal that there is transfer, then my recommendation would be to begin training. Finally, if we develop rules in advance, we will have a systematic basis for the establishment of probes and the selection of sounds for training.

At this point, we conclude our treatment of transfer, even though transfer to conversational speech and transfer to environments outside the clinic have not been discussed. When clinicians speak of the "carryover" problem, they are usually referring to children who either have acquired correct productions but make many errors in conversational speech, or do not make errors in the clinic but do in the classroom and in the home. Their concern is real and demands serious study. Our belief is that the issue of carryover can be best investigated by reference to basic memory processes. For this reason, factors that determine the recall of speech sounds is the theme of our next chapter.

CHAPTER 8

The Retention of Speech Sounds in Conversational Speech

All our efforts to this point are futile if articulatory errors continue to occur in conversational speech in environments away from the clinic. In the classical references, the term *carryover* has come to mean the application of newly learned articulatory responses to conversational speech. It is in this context that the word *automization* has been introduced by Wright, Shelton, and Arndt (1969). To paraphrase the authors, automization refers to correct usage regardless of the speech context and regardless of the environment in which the speaking takes place. The speech context generally subsumes the verbal categories of isolation, syllable, word, phrase, sentence, and conversational speech. The traditional clinical routine is to begin with isolation and continue in the sequential order listed above until mastery in conversation is achieved. At this point training in non-clinical environments is begun.

Elsewhere we have questioned the validity of initiating instruction with phonetic isolation, and, furthermore, we have recommended that training in conversational skill with nonce items should begin before newly learned articulatory responses are introduced into words. Our recommendations for training are outlined below:

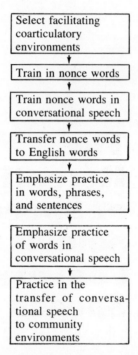

In this chapter procedures for achieving transfer are discussed. The time at which transfer should be implemented is also an important consideration, for which we have few answers. Included in our discussion are a good number of transfer techniques that are currently practiced. Some emphasize parental and teacher intervention while others rely heavily on maintenance strategies.

PERSPECTIVE ON TRANSFER TECHNIQUES

It has been observed by many clinicians and documented by Bankson and Byrne (1972) that a certain amount of transfer takes place without the introduction of structured techniques. Furthermore, comparatively more transfer occurs in environments and circumstances that are similar to those in which clinical training occurred. Bankson and Byrne (1972) found that transfer was greater in the child's school (location not specified by the authors) than in the child's home.

Transfer is very small when the level of initial learning is low, as judged by the findings of Johnston and Johnston (1972). In their study, children were reinforced for correct productions during activity periods, which included story telling, card games, and language arts. Observation of the children during free play activities indicated that correct productions were rarely used. Possibly, more correct productions would have been used in the play period if the children had achieved a high level of proficiency during the activity periods. When the children were later reinforced by their teachers for correct productions during the play periods, the number of correct productions increased dramatically.

Van Riper (1939) has long advocated that transfer should be implemented in environments contiguous to and similar to the clinical environment. In addition, he has recommended that the child's clinician be present when transfer is initiated. Furthermore, the Johnston and Johnston study suggests that transfer will be minimal if the initial level of learning is low unless reinforcement is continued in the non-clinical environments.

CONVERSATIONAL PRINCIPLE 1

Practice in conversation should begin with the child and clinician in environments similar to and near the clinical facility. When sufficient skill is achieved, a second and unfamiliar clinician should be responsible for continuing the dialogues in these same environments.

At this point it is important to introduce another principle, one which is axiomatic to many clinicians. Because transfer may result during word and phrase training, probes of conversational speech should be made.

CONVERSATIONAL PRINCIPLE 2

When a certain level of success is achieved in words and phrases (perhaps after twenty words are well learned), it is recommended that the degree of transfer to conversational speech be assessed. The interval for the probe does not need to extend beyond five or ten minutes. A count should be made of the proportion of instances in which the target sound was said correctly. Weekly or biweekly records should be kept.

Diedrich (1971) advises using a phoneme/minute count of the number of correct sounds. He further recommends charting a child's performance every ten days, in much the same way an economist plots the Dow Jones averages. I believe records should be kept, but Diedrich's elaborate charting procedure is unnecessary. The type of test and the interval between tests would be determined by a number of circumstances, many of which are discussed in this text.

PARENTAL AIDS

At some point we need to concern ourselves with transfer to school, home, and play activities. What role should the parents and teachers play? Our discussion here centers on the parents.

Our knowledge of the influence of parental behavior on articulatory change comes from the important studies of Sommers and his colleagues (Sommers et al., 1959; Sommers, 1962; Sommers et al., 1964). The results of these studies showed that, when parents were informed about articulatory errors in particular and speech errors in general, and were given home assignments to carry out, the rate of articulatory improvement was accelerated. It should be pointed out that, in the investigations of Sommers and his colleagues, articulation was measured in word lists and not in conversational contexts, and so the results do not relate directly to the study of conversational proficiency. However, Bankson and Byrne (1972), Shelton, Johnson, and Arndt (1972), and Wing and Heimgartner (1973) report a small proportion of successful transfer to conversational speech in the home environment. As indicated shortly, the degree of success in the home environment seems to mirror the level of conversational proficiency in the clinic.

The advice given to parents varies somewhat from study to study, but, in the main, it is simply an extension of well accepted clinical practices. The collected advice of the several authors mentioned above can be summarized as follows:

1. The clinician should inform parents about the nature of articulatory errors.
2. The parents should observe clinical sessions.
3. The parents should provide the child with a set of pictures and try to teach each sound.
4. The parents should listen to their child read for a short period each day, at which time praise should be given for correct responses.
5. At some later time, the parents should listen to conversational speech and continue to praise correct articulatory responses.
6. The number of correct responses for reading and conversation should be counted and charted by the parent so that the child can observe his progress.

7. The parents should indicate to their child when a correct response occurs, and they should correct the incorrect responses.

Most of the above practices are not to be recommended as a package to parents. Indeed, when they have been collectively used to teach conversational speech, articulation is somewhat improved, but far less than we would expect even though the training program involved parental tutors (Carrier, 1970; Shelton, Johnson and Arndt, 1972; Wing and Heimgartner, 1973). In retrospect, these practices depart little from the intuitively guided suggestions of the early speech correction authorities.

Why, then, is transfer to conversational speech so unsuccessful? Parental tasks, like those outlined above, apparently serve to "remind" the child that he should use his newly acquired sounds. Therefore, that transfer to conversational speech is unsuccessful cannot be attributed to an absence of stimulus reminders, or, in Skinnerian terminology, that the S^D (discriminative stimulus) is no longer present.

INTERFERENCE

Perhaps we should follow other pursuits. One dimension, which shows promise, relates to the concept of *interference,* competition between the error sound and the newly acquired sound. If the error sound competes vigorously with the standard sound, the effectiveness of cueing, whether given by the parent or the child, will be considerably diminished. Elsewhere we have spelled out interference and how it relates to the recall of speech sounds (Winitz, 1969; Winitz and Bellerose, 1972).

Interference and its effect on memory is a complex issue and currently is very unsettling in the minds of memory theorists (see Winitz and Bellerose, 1969, and Postman and Underwood 1973). Interference can be described in a number of ways. For our purposes, let us assume that it relates primarily to the competition between two responses. If, for example, there are two names for the same object, and one is well learned and one is not, the strong response will dominate the weak response. The term chesterfield is an uncommon significate for the word couch. Having been exposed to this word in no way guarantees recall. Failure to remember may be a function of the fact that the words couch or sofa interfere with the recall of *chesterfield.* We can illustrate the competition as follows:

Learn		*Recall*	
Stimulus	*Response*	*Stimulus*	*Response*
couch (the real object)	chesterfield	couch (the real object)	?

Clinical Example

Interference is also reflected in the recall of speech sounds. Let us assume that a young child learns to say /r/ correctly in words, and, therefore, the clinician begins training in conversation. The traditional approach is simply to provide the child with practice by trumping up a conversation. Soon the clinician realizes that transfer to conversational speech is minimal.

In a great number of cases articulatory errors are reduced after protracted sessions in conversation. Have the articulatory patterns changed because of practice? Perhaps the changes are a result of a reduction in interference.

At the University, in my waggish way, I have always provoked considerable jocularity by demonstrating to college students that they cannot pronounce /t/ and /z/ in sequence. They assure me that they can pronounce these two sounds without any difficulty. Then I ask them to say /bætz/. The /tz/ cluster is mispronounced as either /ts/ or /dz/. Here the interference stems from two permissible sequences, /ts/ and /dz/. In other instances single sounds can also generate interference.

Clinical Example

A young child substitutes /θ/ for /s/. After a series of clinical sessions /s/ is produced correctly in words. As conversation is introduced, the /θ/ seems to return about half the time. Why is transfer to conversation so difficult?

Transfer to conversation seems to be related to the level of articulation proficiency in isolated words and sentences. Two studies were conducted in Ralph Shelton's laboratory, and in one (Wright, Shelton, and Arndt, 1969), transfer to conversational speech lagged behind sound mastery in words. In fact, in this study transfer was unexceptional (about 33%), even after there was almost perfect correction of the error sounds in words. A different result was obtained by Shelton, Johnson, and Arndt (1972). In this second study sound mastery in sentences paralleled that in words. The children in this second study had a higher level of articulation proficiency and also received training from their parents for a four-week period. Another investigator, Diedrich (1971), observed that conversational proficiency begins to develop before there is complete correction of the error sounds in isolated words. However, this fact should not encourage clinicians to begin conversational training prematurely.

In general, as indicated in the preceding pages, when an appraisal of parental assistance was made, the majority of studies indicates that transfer of newly acquired sounds to conversational speech is not something that happens quickly.

Again, our position on this matter is that the error sound competes with the correct sound at time of recall and "blocks" its availability. There is a second explanation. Possibly, the phonetic contexts and syllabic structures are different from those in which the correct sound was trained. This explanation is unlikely, especially if the words and phrases that prefaced conversational training are well learned. We prefer to think that other sentential elements serve as stimuli that elicit the error sound. Speech production, as we have stressed above, is the result of semantic, syntactic, phonological, and phonetic planning. Conversation intensifies these sentential units, and, in turn, increases the likelihood of the error sound being elicited.

The arousal value of the error sound can be mitigated by a clinician, who breaks into the child's sentences and tells him to use the sound correctly. We all know that this practice is difficult and artificial. It is almost impossible for the clinician, or for that matter, any listener, to know when the child will utter his newly acquired sound in running speech. However, the mere presence of the clinician, as well as the clinical environment, can serve to remind the child that he should use his newly acquired sound. On the other hand, a reminding situation is of little value if the newly acquired sound cannot be retrieved from memory. Again, with reference to our previous example, even if one learns to utter /bætz/ he will not do it correctly every time, even if he is reminded to "say it correctly."

In summary, practice is not the modus operandi by which errors in conversational speech can be eliminated. The fact that practice eventually leads to a reduction of errors means that certain sentential stimuli no longer elicit errors. How this comes about is, at this time, open to question. Most likely it can be explained as an instance of transfer similar in many respects to the syllable-word transfer discussed above. Those cues that elicit the correct sound in isolated words and phrases will continue to operate in conversational speech. An error produced in conversational speech means that there are competing stimuli that are greater in strength than those for the isolated words and phrases. At this time a clinical example may be helpful.

Clinical Example

Let us assume that, with training, a young child no longer substitutes /θ/ for /s/. He can produce /s/ correctly in a great number of words and phrases.

For example, not only can he say "soup" correctly, but he also can say "hot soup" correctly.

Assume now that the teacher engages him in conversational speech that leads to the child uttering, "I was cold and so I went home and mother made me a cup of hot soup." The child knew from the very beginning that he was going to talk about soup, for semantic ideas precede syntactic operations. All of the many stimuli preceding the word soup are much greater in number than the stimuli present in the words hot and soup. There may be other instances in which the sentential cues are weaker than those learned for words and phrases. For example, a child's response to his mother's question, "Do you want juice or soup?," might be "I want soup" or "Give me soup." The latter two sentences may elicit a correct /s/ and, by generalization, transfer to sentences like "I think I want soup." In time, there should be generalization to a variety of sentences types.

As yet there is no evidence to support the above speculations. It would be interesting to initiate a series of investigations, which would examine sentence length, and syntactic and semantic intentions, as they relate to articulatory errors. Semantic intention might be measured in terms of the number of words between the introduction of an idea or concept and its expression. If, for example, we are examining /s/ we could develop a conversation with a child and note the occurrence of each word that begins with /s/. We would then count the number of words, admittedly a gross measure, between the introduction of the concept and the child's utterance of the particular word beginning with /s/.

An illustration of this word count procedure would be helpful. Let us assume the following dialogue takes place between the clinician and the child:

Clinician: It's sure cold today.
Child: Yes, it makes me feel chilly all over.
Clinician: You know it would be good to have something *hot* for lunch.
Child: I love to eat tomato *soup* when I'm cold.

The word count begins with *hot* and terminates with *soup,* giving a word count of seven; that is, seven words intervene between the words hot and soup.

If there is a relation between semantic intention, as defined by the above proposed word count index, and frequency of articulatory errors, careful consideration should be given to the design of sentences when conversational practice is emphasized. At first, sentences should be developed in which the semantic intention is a few short words away from the practice word. Later the interval between the semantic intention and the practice word should be increased. Examples of progressively larger semantic units are:

1. What goes in here? (Show the child a soup bowl.)
2. What is hot and goes in here? (Show the child a soup bowl.)
3. This is a tomato. Lots of foods come from tomatoes. Tell me, do you like tomatoes, and what are some of the foods we use tomatoes for? (Show the child a soup bowl.)

Until further research is conducted, we will make no attempt to offer a principle at this time. If forthcoming research is supportive, however, then the development of conversational protocols, which maximize generalization, is an endeavor that should be encouraged.

SELF-TRAINING

We now return to the question of cueing. As discussed earlier, several investigators have recommended that parents should play a major role in the implementation of carryover. Much of this is speculation, however, because in two studies (Bankson and Byrne, 1972; Shelton, Johnson, and Arndt, 1972) conversational proficiency in the home reflected that achieved in the clinic. The inference is clear: The role of the parents seems to be relatively minor in the implementation of conversational proficiency in the home, especially if conversational proficiency is not achieved in the clinic.

At this point, we should emphasize that this conclusion pertains only to conversational transfer and not to the acquisition of sounds. As indicated above, Sommers and his colleagues have presented sufficient evidence to indicate that mothers can assist clinicians in the early stages of articulatory training. Mothers also can assist in the maintenance of conversational skills. It is unlikely, however, that mothers can teach conversational proficiency. Although we have little evidence to support our claim, it is our contention that carryover to environments outside the clinic can be achieved quickly and easily once conversational proficiency is reached in the clinic and in the immediate surroundings. Others may not hold this point of view.

Self-Cueing

A procedure that emphasizes self-cueing has been proposed by Diedrich (1971). Self-cueing can be used for two purposes: to assist in the transfer process, and to maintain a level of achievement, either between clinic sessions or at the conclusion of clinical training.

Self-cueing refers to a procedure by which an individual monitors his own production. Diedrich (1971) outlines three parts to this process: explanation, demonstration, and practice.

Initially, the clinician explains that the goal of speech training is to learn to use the ''target'' sound in conversational speech. Next, two counters are provided to the child. The clinician demonstrates how to use the counters. The child is to press one when he utters the sound correctly and to press the other when he utters the sound incorrectly. A stop watch is also provided in the event the same time base is to be used on each day. Finally, the child is given practice with all of these paraphernalia.

Essentially there are two practice steps. First, the child converses with the clinician and counts correct and incorrect responses. After each response the clinician and child confer to determine the reliability of the child's decision. If the child's decision is incorrect (that is, if the child calls a correct response wrong or an incorrect response right) the clinician and the child confer further. At this point, the clinician instructs the child on how to evaluate correct and incorrect responses. If, however, the child's response is in agreement with the clinician, he is handsomely praised. Second, the child is asked to record his responses for certain periods of the day in the home or in the school environment. He is also taught to chart his responses; he is given paper to plot the number of correct responses per day or per week. The chart serves as a focus for discussion at the next clinical session.

The recording of one's own articulation can be regarded as a variety of self-cueing. There is a preliminary study that seems to recommend the use of self-cueing. Johnston and Johnston (1972) reported the findings of an experiment in which children were taught to count correct responses. The counting took place in the classroom, during which time the teacher also counted correct responses. Although the number of correct responses increased, it is difficult to determine whether or not it was the result of self-counting. During the period of time that the subjects were counting their own correct responses, the teacher was also ''correcting'' incorrect sounds. An example of a corrective statement was ''No, Johnny, fish not pish.''

If transfer is initiated before conversational proficiency, self-cueing probably will be of little value, as Johnston and Johnston (1972) found. In that study, self-cueing was successful when it was carefully monitored in activity periods, but there was little transfer when subjects were given counters and told to count in play periods. Apparently, the error sounds had not been extinguished fully in the activity periods, suggesting that the introduction of self-cueing was premature.

Self-evaluation as a clinical technique needs thorough testing. There are many procedures that can be developed and submitted for experimental study (Webb and Siegenthaler, 1957). One that is often practiced is joint evaluation. Here the child and clinician compare and discuss each production. Presumably, this technique is to encourage the evaluation of target sounds subsequent to their production.

Paired-Stimuli Technique

Recently, a new approach for teaching the acquisition and recall of sounds has been developed. Called the paired-stimuli technique, it involves an interesting departure from traditional generalization tasks. Unlike the classical approaches (e.g., Van Riper, 1939; McDonald, 1964; and Winitz, 1969), in which imitation is used, the paired-stimuli technique emphasizes retrieval from memory as a procedure for teaching sounds.

In the Weston and Irwin approach, the correct production of a sound is paired with an incorrect production. A word is selected in which the test phoneme is said correctly; this is called the *key* word. Several additional words are selected in which the test phoneme is said incorrectly; these words are called *training* words. First, the subject pronounces the key word, and then he is asked to pronounce a training word. Using this procedure (pairing a key word with training words), Weston and Irwin (1971) and Irwin and Griffith (1973) found that subjects were able to transfer the correct sound of key words to the appropriate training words. However, neither study compared the efficiency of this procedure with the more traditional practice of imitation (e.g., Powell and McReynolds, 1969). Therefore, it is difficult to know whether or not emphasis on self-production results in an increase in efficiency.

An interesting aspect of the paired-stimuli technique is that it requires the target sound, which is an element of the key word, to be retrieved from memory. In the imitation technique, auditory stimulation is provided and the demand on memory is short-term. To emphasize the heavy emphasis on memory required of subjects taught by the paired stimuli-technique, the term *self-retrieval* is introduced.

The Weston and Irwin procedure was originally developed to facilitate acquisition, but recently (Weston and Irwin, 1973) it has been modified to include practice with key words and training words in sentences. Practice with sentences is included because Weston and Irwin contend that recall ("carryover") is enhanced.

Self-Retrieval

We turn now to a discussion of self-retrieval and retention. Self-retrieval is a frequent practice of some speech pathologists who believe it is a significant element in gaining transfer to conversational speech. The procedure works this way. After a child can correctly imitate the standard sound, he is given intensive practice with pictorial stimuli. The reason for using pictures is to assure that the subject will learn to self-elicit the target sound.

Let us assume that a child with a θ/s substitution learns to articulate correctly the /s/ in a variety of phonetic and grammatical contexts. However, he continues to misarticulate the /s/ in conversation.

The clinician then arranges a series of pictures in front of the child and asks him to name each picture. The pictures are designed to elicit the /s/ in a variety of linguistic environments. If the child misarticulates the /s/ sound, the clinician usually pronounces the word and then asks the child to repeat the utterance.

The sound production task described in the investigations of Shelton and his colleagues (1972) indicates fairly strongly that the ability to self-retrieve is a consequence of imitation training. Furthermore, the Shelton investigation, as well as the Bankson and Byrne (1972) study, suggests that conversational proficiency reflects the level of success during imitation training. There seems to be no need to require an intervening level of training, which in this context we call self-retrieval. Essentially, this is the approach taken by Winitz and Reeds (1975) in their second language program. Students are taught to comprehend the second language, not to speak it or read it. The evidence, as summarized by Winitz and Reeds (1975), is very convincing: Children acquire mastery of language not by practice in production, but by being able to comprehend the language they hear.

Does training in pronouncing the sound when a picture is presented (self-retrieval training) facilitate recall? In a recent study, Winitz and Bellerose (in press) found that self-retrieved responses did not facilitate recall. In that study the subjects learned through imitation training to pronounce the non-English sound /ç/ in nonce words. After mastery was achieved, the imitation groups continued to receive imitation training. The self-retrieval groups were instructed to say the sound from memory. There was no difference between the groups when, five days later, they were asked to recall the /ç/ sound. At this time, our conjecture is that the auditory "image" is primary. Fluency in the *recall* of productions is apparently a consequence of a high degree of auditory training. After all, if the auditory image is well implanted, production should follow easily.

The above discussion should not lead us to conclude that imitative and spontaneous utterances are reflections of the same underlying process. It would be absurd to suggest that they are. When a sound has not been acquired, a correct, imitative response can involve only short-term memory. The subject hears the word or phrase and is asked to repeat it almost immediately. If more than five to ten seconds elapse, there will be decay in short-term memory, and, at this point, an imitative response will be equivalent to one elicited by a picture. In other words, imitation and pictorial elicitation are thought to be equivalent when short-term memory is ruled out.

Memory theorists seem to think that interference will produce decrements in recall in both short-term and long-term memory. Therefore, when interference is relatively weak, that is, when the error sound and the standard sound are equally available to the subject, immediate imitation should produce more correct responses than pictorial elicitation. The auditory stimulus simply indicates the correct alternative. When the interval for eliciting imitation exceeds short-term memory, errors that result as a function of interference should be equivalent for imitation and pictorial elicitation.

There is at least partial substantiation for the above speculations. In one investigation, Winitz and Bellerose (1972) trained young children to learn a series of non-English clusters, namely /zn, ʃn, zm, zw, ʃw/. All of the clusters were learned as substitute responses for the word snow. Thus, a child learning the cluster /zn/ learned to say /znow/ when a picture of snow was presented. Seven days later the subjects were tested for recall. Imitation was examined by having the subjects repeat tape-recorded utterances; self-retrieval was examined by showing the subject a picture of snow and asking him to pronounce it in "the way you learned it." Imitative recall was markedly superior to pictorial recall.

Pictorial recall reflects most closely the factors at work during conversational speech. A subject who can imitate correctly, but who responds incorrectly to pictures or makes an error in conversation, has the requisite phonetic skills for producing the standard sound. Non-imitative errors presumably reflect an inability to *retrieve* the correct sound, not an inability to *make* the sound. An inability to self-retrieve is presumably caused by competition from the error sound at the time of recall.

Perhaps we have taken a circuitous route to make judgmental claims about interference. If, however, we accept the premise that transfer to conversational speech will not be well effected until competition from the error sound is reduced, then it seems clear that practice in conversation only indirectly accomplishes our goal. Somehow embedded within the methodology of conversational practice is an underlying process that reduces interference. The explanation we gave above was that there is generalization from stimuli less likely to elicit the error sound, to stimuli that provoke the error sound.

Our next step is to determine how to accelerate generalization so as to reduce elicitation of the error sound. Before suggesting a procedure, which has yet to be researched, we should first report another finding of the Winitz and Bellerose (1972) study.

In the Winitz and Bellerose (1972) investigation, which involved the learning of non-English clusters as substitute responses for /sn/ in the word snow, it was found that phonetic similarity governed the amount of recall when the response was pictorially elicited. For example, /zn/ is more similar to /sn/ than is /zm/. Also /ʃn/ is much more similar to /sn/ than is /zw/. The more similar the two clusters, the greater the recall, as instanced by the fact that /zn/ produced better recall than /zm/, and /ʃn/ produced better recall than /zw/. Recall for /ʃn/ and /zm/ was about the same. Apparently, the error sound may at times facilitate recall by mediating between the significate and the standard pronunciation.

Generalization: Clinical Example

A young child substitutes /b/ for /v/. He soon learns to utter correctly words containing /v/, such as valentine, vegetable, and avenue. When conversational training begins, the child seems to regress; *v*'s are pronounced as *b*'s. One clinical approach would be to begin conversational training by emphasizing generalization, as indicated above. Another approach would be to make /b/ a link in the chain that eventuates in the production of /v/.

Below is what is referred to as a mediation paradigm. The sign is *valentine,* either as a thought process or as an object:

Sign or thought process	*Implicit response*	*External response*

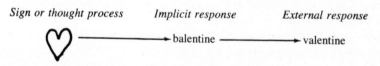

As conversational training begins, the sign *valentine* elicits the production *balentine*. With time and the proper generalization training, *balentine* will yield to *valentine*.

There is probably more to it than simply a reduction in the response strength of the error sound, or, in the above case, /b/ yielding to /v/.

Because the subject has been instructed to say /v/ in place of /b/, the two sounds become associated in the context of words containing /v/. We conjecture that /b/ will compete with /v/ early in training, but in time /b/ will serve as an elicitor of /v/.

Our hunch is that the associative link between the error sound and the correct sound is a critical component in gaining conversational fluency. And, if it is, we should favor its employ.

It could be no other way. When a young child is instructed to learn to say correctly the word valentine, he knows that /vælɛntaɪn/ is merely a substitute for /bælɛtaɪn/. It is like the school teacher who comes West. When she hears the word chalkboard she knows this word is another name for blackboard. She also realizes that sack is another name for bag. The Easterner who settles in Chicago knows that /ʃɪkagoʊ/ is pronounced /ʃɪkɔgoʊ/, and, if the social pressures are such, may replace /a/ with /ɔ/. The /a/ competes with /ɔ/, but eventually these two sounds become associated for the recently settled Chicagoan.

In much the same way, an association also develops between the error sound and the target sound. When it no longer serves as a mediator, the error sound drops out.

If we accept the premise of the above argument—that the error sound serves to elicit, either covertly or overtly, the standard sound—our training regimen should include procedures to strengthen this association.

We propose the following to strengthen the link between /b/ and /v/ after /v/ has been mastered in words and phrases. The subject first hears the incorrect pronunciation and is asked to respond with the correct pronunciation:

Stimulus (The child hears the words pronounced incorrectly.)	*Response* (The child pronounces the words correctly.)
1. balentine	valentine
2. begetable	vegetable
3. abenue	avenue

Many trials of "incorrect-incorrect" pairings should be presented to the child. Unlike negative practice, the child never pronounces the words incorrectly. In negative practice (Van Riper, 1972) incorrect productions are practiced because it is believed that a child who corrected his error should once again experience the contrast between the correct production and the incorrect production. The validity of negative practice has never been tested.

With the technique recommended above, the child hears only the incorrect pronunciation but responds with the correct pronunciation. Children can learn this association easily. The end result of this training is to provoke the association between the error sound and the correct sound so that, in conversational speech, the likelihood of self-correction becomes increased. A child might be heard to say, "I want a balen—valentine."

CHAPTER 9

The Articulation Test: A Second Look

At this time, it would seem instructive to bend our way back through these several chapters. We have covered material relevant to the many dimensions of articulatory training. Our segmentation of training has led to the several general categories: discrimination, production, transfer, and retention. Each of these areas requires specialized testing procedures.

Counter to the prevailing mood, we have argued that the initial articulation testing program should be linked to behavioral goals. Our initial task is to determine which sounds are in error, and we have suggested that we can gather this information by examining conversational speech. From there we can test our hypotheses with isolated word lists, making use of any one of a number of commercially available test kits.

It should be clear from the outset that we should not be guided by the format of articulation tests. Rather, we should frame an initial hypothesis and test it out.

ARTICULATORY TRAINING

Clinical Example

Let us assume for the moment that we have examined a young child and found that the /s/ and /z/ sounds are produced incorrectly in conversation.

We might ask the following questions:

1. Are the /s/ and /z/ sounds produced incorrectly in isolated words?
2. What is the degree of consistency of the articulation errors?
3. What are the phonetic substitutions? (Distortions are regarded as substitutions in the analysis.) The errors should be transcribed precisely, and the missing phonetic features should be noted.
4. Are the missing distinctive features available in the sounds the child produces correctly?
5. Can the child produce the sound when an auditory representation is provided by the clinician?
6. Are there underlying rules that jointly account for the mispronunciation of /z/ and /s/? Frame a rule and test it out by examining additional words and phonetic contexts.
7. Finally, what is the child's discrimination between /z/ and the error sound, and between /s/ and the error sound?

With all of the above information, a program of articulatory training can be tentatively established. The testing, however, never ends. As we frame hypotheses about phonetic context and phonological rules, we need to test our assumptions. As we examine transfer, probe tests must be administered. It seems that our principles guide our clinical routines, and sophisticated testing will have a strong influence on our choice of clinical routines.

Relationship of Hypotheses to Methodology

In this short book we have examined methodological principles underlying the treatment procedures of articulatory disorders. Our review has taken us into areas that are generally regarded as traditional ones. However, something new has been added. Phonological theory and the psychology of learning are the elements we use to sculpt new methodologies. As we mix these new raw materials, additional hypotheses will form.

Our pretesting should reflect these insights. Stated in another way, articulatory testing should be used to examine performance; it should not constrain our methodological procedures. The behaviors we test must be those which our methodological approaches direct us to examine. Our testing will provide us with new data to be sifted and strained. After careful analysis, behavioral regimens will be written. As with every endeavor, there will be need for constant reevaluation and appraisal. It seems, then, that articulation testing will continue as long as there is need for clinical instruction, and the frequency of testing will depend on our willingness to examine clinical hypotheses.

SUMMARY OF THE CLINICAL PROCESS

At this point the instructional models that we have discussed can be presented in summary form. For illustrative purposes we can refer to Figure 9.1.

The first step is the important one. We use, as indicated in Figure 9.1, a testing procedure to shape our program of instruction. We listen to conversational speech and frame an hypothesis about the child's speech errors.

Using standard pictorial articulation tests, we examine a great number of phonetic contexts and linguistic environments. We determine what phonetic features appear in the child's sound repertoire. Furthermore, we need to determine if the child can make the standard sounds when stimulated (stimulability). Finally, we inspect the data carefully to determine the underlying rules that govern sets of sounds. This analysis is difficult, requiring considerable training beyond the introductory articulation course.

At this point we are ready to look at the discrimination process. The research findings tell us that we should be concerned only with sounds that are in error. A discerning ear is critical at this point. Identification of the error sound should be made with certainty by the clinician.

Once the error sound is established, a paired-comparison discrimination program can be established. For example, the phonetic errors for /s/ are usually a frontal lisp, a [θ] or [t̪]; a lateral lisp, a voiceless [l], denoted [l̥], or a voiceless fricative [l], denoted [ɬ]; a back fricative, usually [ʃ]; and sometimes a retroflex [s], denoted [ş]. For each phonetic context the error sound and the standard sound are compared. Discrimination learning can be taught rapidly and efficiently if the clinician makes use of the methodology of distinctive stimulus pretraining, as discussed in Chapter 4.

After discrimination training, acquisition principles are applied. If the "phoneme," or a variant (allophone) of the phoneme is available, discrimination training would seem to be unimportant. However, we would recommend testing discrimination before concluding that training in this dimension is unessential. There is the possibility that, for some children, stimulability may not be correlated with discrimination. It seems to be an unlikely fact, but the important evidence has not yet been provided.

Acquisition can be facilitated by making use of nonce words and by ascertaining which units facilitate right to left coarticulation. After we take cognizance of the fact that sounds are usually produced correctly in at least some contexts, our search for facilitating sequences will be that much easier. If, for example, an /s/ sound is produced correctly preceding a /t/, we would concentrate on other post-*s* alveolar contexts, such as /sn/, /sl/, and so forth. In addition, vocalic environments would be varied.

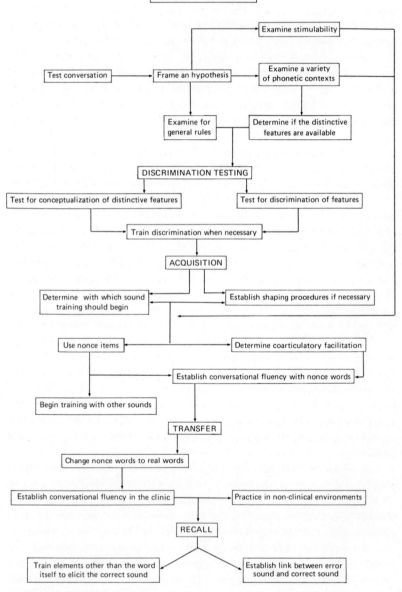

Figure 9.1. A block diagram of the clinical process of articulatory training.

Skillfully, the clinician teaches the child to accept nonce words as real objects. Gradually, nonce items are introduced into sentences. Eventually, the child will gain fluency with these words; they will no longer be the fanciful fantasies of the clinician, but the realities of the child.

When complete fluency is developed with about twenty nonce items, real words are introduced. Initially the phonemes of the nonce items are discarded, and ideally the by-product forms real words, e.g., /irdʌgə/ becomes /ir/, /irɪb/ becomes /rɪb/, and /istim/ becomes /ist/ and /stim/. After this exercise is completed, the usual lists of English words can be used for training.

As new words are introduced, all of the mechanisms of transfer are brought into focus. The use of English words, phonetic variants, word position, and other phonetic contexts and sentential units must be reckoned with. Full use of transfer paradigms should be made. The terminal goal at this point is conversational fluency in the clinic.

Experience with conversational units outside the clinic is not to be ignored, although the evidence now suggests that, in most instances, there will be maximal transfer to non-clinical environments when complete fluency is established in the clinic. At this point, it is most critical to survey the child's articulation behavior. Our survey will tell us whether or not fluency has transferred to the classroom or to the home. Testing of transfer beyond the clinic is not easy, but, as we have suggested, it can be done.

To assist the child as he enters new environments, we have recommended conversational training and strengthening of the associative link between the error sound and the standard sound. Again, it is important to recognize that there should be constant reevaluation of the many and varied training procedures. If, for example, associative training between the stimulus of the error sound and the standard sound does not affect transfer, this training should be discontinued. Of course, it should be given a fair chance.

Articulation testing is regarded as a procedure for examining output. Careful description and analysis at critical points in the clinical experience of a client is important if progress is to be evaluated. On the basis of testing, revisions are made in the clinical program. When to test is a clinical decision; it directly reflects the program of instruction. Once again, it is important to state that the use of commercially available tests can transfer able clinicians into sterile performers. The clinician should select those tests that add precision to the evaluation process. The tests should not govern the performance of the clinician. This danger always remains because test makers often do not realize the complexity of the clinical processes, as outlined in Figure 9.1.

Finally a word of caution. The block diagrams presented in Figure 9.1 are derived from the known facts, as interpreted by this author. Although the schema may seem complete, there are no padlocks. It is our professional responsibility to respect change. What is inscribed above is only a galley proof. As you are reading this text, scholars are rubbing out paragraphs and making notes in the margin.

There is an old story of the two Wandering Jews who argued about the pronunciation of the word light. One argued forcefully that it was *dos licht* the other *dos lecht*. The first friend tried to resolve the problem by finding a dictionary on Yiddish pronunciations. Fortunately for him, the volume recommended *dos licht*. He turned to his friend and said, "See, *dos licht* is correct; it says so right here."

Literature Cited

Abbs, M. S., and F. D. Minifie. 1969. Effect of acoustic cues in fricatives on perceptual confusions in preschool children. J. Acoust. Soc. Amer. 46: 1535—1542.

Ainsworth, S. 1948. Speech Correction Methods. Prentice-Hall, Englewood Cliffs, N.J.

Albright, R. W., and J. B. Albright. 1958. Application of descriptive linguistics to child language. J. Speech Hear. Res. 1: 257–261.

Ali, L., T. Gallagher, J. Goldstein, and R. Daniloff. 1971. Perception of coarticulated nasality. J. Acoust. Soc. Amer. 49: 538–540.

Applegate, J. R. 1961. Phonological rules of a subdialect of English. Word 17: 186–193.

Bankson, N. W., and M. C. Byrne. 1972. The effect of a timed correct sound production task on carryover. J. Speech Hear. Res. 15: 160–168.

Brown, R., C. Cazden, and U. Bellugi. 1969. The child's grammar from I to III. In J. P. Hill (ed.), Minnesota Symposia on Child Psychology. Vol. 2. Minneapolis Minnesota Press, Minneapolis.

Bullowa, M., L. G. Jones, and A. R. Duckert. 1964. The acquisition of a word. Lang. Speech 7: 107–111.

Cairns, H. S., and F. Williams. 1972. An analysis of the substitution errors of a group of standard English-speaking children. J. Speech Hear. Res. 15: 811–820.

Carrier, J. K. 1970. A program of articulation therapy administered by mothers. J. Speech Hear. Disord. 35: 344–353.

Catford, J. C., and P. Ladefoged. 1968. Practical Phonetic Exercises. Working Papers in Phonetics, UCLA.

Chao, Y. R. 1968. Language and Symbolic Systems. Cambridge University Press, London.

Chomsky, N., and M. Halle. 1968. The Sound Pattern of English. Harper & Row, New York.

Compton, A. 1970. Generative studies of children's phonological disorders. J. Speech Hear. Disord. 35: 315–339.

Curtis, J. F. 1970. Segmenting the stream of speech. In J. Griffith and L. E. Miner (eds.), The First Lincolnland Conference on Dialectology. University of Alabama Press, University, Ala.

Curtis, J. R., and J. C. Hardy. 1959. A phonetic study of misarticulation of /r/. J. Speech Hear. Res. 2: 244–257.

Daniloff, R. G., and R. E. Hammarberg. 1973. On defining coarticulation. J. Phonet. 1: 239–248.

Daniloff, R. G., and K. Moll. 1968. Coarticulation of lip rounding. J. Speech Hear. Res. 11: 707–721.

Diedrich, W. M. 1971. Procedures for counting and charting a target phoneme. Lang. Speech Hear. Serv. Schools No. 5: 18–32.

Eimas, P. D., E. R. Siqueland, P. Jusczyk, and J. Vigorito. 1971. Speech perception in infants. Science 171: 303–306.

Elbert, M., R. L. Shelton, and W. B. Arndt. 1967. A task for evaluation of articulation change. I. Development of methodology. J. Speech Hear. Res. 10: 281–288.

Faircloth, M. A., and S. R. Faircloth. 1970. An analysis of the articulatory behavior of a speech-defective child in connected speech and in isolated-word responses. J. Speech Hear. Disord. 35: 51–61.

Gerber, A. 1973. Goal: Carryover. Temple University Press, Philadelphia.

Haas, W. 1963. Phonological analysis of a case of dyslalia. J. Speech Hear. Disord. 28: 239–246.

Halle, M. 1964a. On the basis of phonology. In J. A. Fodor and J. J. Katz (eds.), The Structure of Language. Prentice-Hall, Englewood Cliffs, N.J.

Halle, M. 1964b. Phonology in generative grammar. In J. A. Fodor and J. J. Katz (eds.), The Structure of Language. Prentice-Hall, Englewood Cliffs, N.J.

Henke, W. L. 1967. Preliminaries to speech analysis based upon an articulatory model. Conference Report, 1967 conference on Speech Communication Process, pp. 170–177. A. F. Cambridge Research Laboratory, Cambridge, Mass.

House, A. S. 1961. Letter to the editor. J. Speech Hear. Res. 4: 194–197.

Irwin, J. V., and F. A. Griffith. 1973. A theoretical and operational analysis of the paired stimuli technique. In W. D. Wolfe and D. J. Goulding (eds.), Articulation and Learning. Charles C Thomas, Springfield, Ill.

Jakobson, R., C. Fant, and M. Halle. 1952. Preliminaries to Speech Analysis. MIT Press, Cambridge, Mass.

Johnston, J. M., and G. T. Johnston. 1972. Modification of consonant speech-sound articulation in young children. J. Appl. Behav. Anal. 5: 233–246.

Kalikow, D. N., and J. A. Swets. 1972. Experiments with computer-controlled displays in second-language learning. IEEE Trans. Audio Electroacoust. 20: 23–28.

Kent, R. D., P. J. Carney, and L. R. Severeid. 1974. Velar movement and timing: Evaluation of a model for binary control. J. Speech Hear. Res. 17: 470–488.

Kent, R. D., and K. L. Moll. 1972. Cinefluorographic analysis of selected lingual consonants. J. Speech Hear. Res. 15: 453–473.

Kozhevnikov, V., and L. Chistovich. 1965. Speech: Articulation and Perception. Translated from the Russian, U.S. Department of Commerce, Washington, D.C.

Ladefoged, P. 1971. Preliminaries to Linguistic Phonetics. University of Chicago Press, Chicago.

Lane, H. 1968. Research on second-language learning. In S. Rosenberg and J. Koplin (eds.), Developments in Applied Psycholinguistic Research. Macmillan, New York.

LaRiviere, C., H. Winitz, J. Reeds, and E. Herriman. 1974. The conceptual reality of selected distinctive features. J. Speech Hear. Res. 17: 122–133.

Leonard, L. B. 1973. Referential effects on articulatory learning. Lang. Speech 16: 45–56.

Lewis, M. M. 1951. Infant Speech: A Study of the Beginning of Language. Humanities Press, New York.

Liberman, A. M., F. S. Cooper, D. P. Shankweiler, and M. Studdert-Kennedy. 1967. Perception of the speech code. Psychol. Rev. 74: 431–461.

Lisker, L., and A. S. Abramson. 1964. A cross-language study of voicing in initial stops: Acoustic measurements. Word 10: 384–422.

McDonald, E. T. 1964. Articulation Testing and Treatment: A Sensory Motor Approach. Stanwix House, Pittsburgh.

McNutt, J. C., and R. A. Keenan. 1970. Comment on "The relationship between articulatory deficits and syntax in speech defective children." J. Speech Hear. Res. 13: 666–667.

McReynolds, L. V. 1972. Articulation generalization during articulation training. Lang. Speech 15: 149–155.

McReynolds, L. V., and S. Bennett, 1972. Distinctive feature generalization in articulation training. J. Speech Hear. Disord. 37: 462–470.

McReynolds, L. V., and D. L. Engmann. 1975. Distinctive Feature Analysis of Misarticulations. University Park Press, Baltimore.

McReynolds, L. V., and K. Huston. 1971. A distinctive feature analysis of children's misarticulations. J. Speech Hear. Disord. 36: 155–166.

Milisen, R. 1954. A rationale for articulation disorders. J. Speech Hear. Disord. Monogr. Suppl. 4: 6–17.

Moskowitz, A. 1972. Review of Winitz' "Articulatory acquisition and behavior." Language 48: 487–498.

Netsell, R., and B. Daniel. 1974. Neural and mechanical response time for speech production. J. Speech Hear. Res. 17: 608–618.

Pollack, E., and N. S. Rees. 1972. Disorders of articulation: Some clinical applications of distinctive feature theory. J. Speech Hear. Disord. 37: 451–470.

Postman, L., and B. J. Underwood. 1973. Critical issues in interference theory. Memory Cognit. 1:19–40.

Powell, J., and L. V. McReynolds. 1969. A procedure for testing position generalization from articulation training. J. Speech Hear. Res. 3: 629–645.

Powers, M. H. 1971. Functional disorders of articulation: Symptomatology and Etiology. In L. E. Travis (ed.), Handbook of Speech Pathology and Audiology. Appleton-Century-Crofts, New York.

Sapir, S. G. 1972. Auditory discrimination with words and nonsense syllables. Academ. Ther. 7: 307–313.

Salus, P. H., and M. W. Salus. 1974. Developmental neurophysiology and phonological acquisition order. Language 50: 151–160.

Shelton, R. L., M. Elbert, and W. B. Arndt. 1967. A task for evaluation of articulation change. II. Comparison of task scores during baseline and lesson series testing. J. Speech Hear. Res. 10: 578–585.

Shelton, R. L., A. F. Johnson, and W. Arndt. 1972. Monitoring and reinforcement by parents as a means of automating articulatory responses. Percep. Motor Skills 35: 759–767.

Shriner, T. H., and R. G. Daniloff. 1971. Reply to "Comments on the relationship between articulatory deficits and syntax in speech defective children." J. Speech Hear. Res. 14: 442–444.

Shriner, T. H., M. S. Holloway, and R. G. Daniloff. 1969. The relationship between articulatory deficits and syntax in speech defective children. J. Speech Hear. Res. 12: 319–325.

Siegel, G. M., H. Winitz, and H. Conkey. 1963. The influence of testing instrument on articulatory responses of children. J. Speech Hear. Disord. 28: 67–76.

Singh, S. Distinctive Features: Theory and Validation. University Park Press, Baltimore. In press.

Singh, S., and D. C. Frank. 1972. A distinctive feature analysis of the consonantal substitution pattern. Lang. Speech 15: 209–218.

Singh, S., and S. B. Polen, 1972. Use of a distinctive feature model in speech pathology. Acta Symbol. 3: 17–25.

Skinner, B. F. 1938. The Behavior of Organisms. Appleton-Century-Crofts, New York.

Smith, M. W. and S. Ainsworth. 1967. The effects of three types of stimulation on articulatory responses of speech defective children. J. Speech Hear. Res. 10: 333–338.

Smith, N. 1973. The Acquisition of Phonology. Cambridge University Press, London.

Sommers, R. K. 1962. Factors in the effectiveness of mothers trained to aid in speech correction. J. Speech Hear. Disord. 27: 178–186.

Sommers, R. K., A. K. Furlong, F. E. Rhodes, G. R. Fichter, D. C. Bowser, F. G. Copetas, and Z. G. Saunders. 1964. Effects of maternal attitude upon improvement in articulation when mothers are trained to assist in speech correction. J. Speech Hear. Disord. 29: 126–132.

Sommers, R. K., S. P. Shilling, C. D. Paul, F. G. Copetas, D. C. Bowser, and C. J. McClintock. 1959. Training parents of children with functional misarticulation. J. Speech Hear. Res. 2: 258–265.

Spriestersbach, D. C., and J. F. Curtis. 1951. Misarticulation and discrimination of speech sounds. Q. J. Speech 37: 483–491.

Stevens, K. N., A. S. House, and A. P. Paul. 1966. Acoustic description of syllabic nuclei: An interpretation in terms of a dynamic model of articulation. J. Acoust. Soc. Amer. 40: 123–132.

Templin, M. 1957. Certain Language Skills in Children. Institute of Child Welfare Monograph No. 26. University of Minnesota Press, Minneapolis.

Van Riper, C. 1939. Speech Correction: Principles and Methods. Prentice-Hall, Englewood Cliffs, N.J. (Reprinted: 1947, 1972).

Van Riper, C., and J. V. Irwin. 1958. Voice and Articulation. Prentice-Hall, Englewood Cliffs, N.J.

Walsh, H. 1974. On certain practical inadequacies of distinctive feature systems. J. Speech Hear. Disord. 39: 32–43.

Webb, C. E., and B. W. Siegenthaler. 1957. Comparison of aural stimulation methods for teaching speech sounds. J. Speech Hear. Disord. 22: 264–270.

Weber, J. 1970. Patterning of deviant articulation behavior. J. Speech Hear. Disord. 35: 135–141.

Wepman, J. M. 1958. Auditory Discrimination Test: Manual of Directions. Language Research Associates, Chicago.

Weston, A. J., and J. V. Irwin. 1971. Use of paired stimuli in modification of articulation. Percept. Motor Skills 32: 947–957.

Weston, A. J. and J. V. Irwin. 1973. Paired stimuli: Rationale and data. Paper presented at the ASHA Southeastern Regional Conference, Atlanta, May 10, 1973.

Wicklegren, W. A. 1969. Context sensitive coding, associative memory and serial order in (speech) behavior. Psychol. Rev. 76: 1–15.

Wing, D. M., and L. M. Heimgartner. 1973. Articulation carryover procedure implemented by parents. Lang. Speech Hear. Serv. Schools 4: 182–195.

Winitz, H. 1969. Articulatory Acquisition and Behavior. Appleton-Century-Crofts, New York.

Winitz, H., and B. Bellerose. 1965. Phoneme cluster learning as a function of instructional method and age. J. Verb. Learn. Verb. Behav. 4: 98–102.

Winitz, H., and B. Bellerose. 1967. Relation between sound discrimination and sound learning. J. Commun. Disord. 1: 215–235.

Winitz, H., and B. Bellerose. 1972. Effect of similarity of sound substitutions on retention. J. Speech Hear. Res. 15: 677–689.

Winitz, H., and B. Bellerose. Self-retrieval and articulatory retention. J. Speech Hear. Res. 18. In press.

Winitz, H., and O. C. Irwin. 1958. Syllabic and phonetic structure of infants early words. J. Speech Hear. Res. 1: 250–256.

Winitz, H., and L. Preisler. 1965. Discrimination pretraining and sound learning. Percep. Motor Skills 20: 905–916.

Winitz, H., and J. Reeds. 1975. Comprehension and Problem Solving as Strategies for Language Learning. Mouton, The Hague, Netherlands.

Winitz, H., M. E. Scheib, and J. A. Reeds. 1973. Identification of stops and vowels for the burst portion of /p, t, k/ isolated from conversational speech. J. Acoust. Soc. Amer. 51: 1309–1317.

Wright, V., R. L. Shelton, and W. B. Arndt. 1969. A task for evaluation of articulation change. III. Imitative task scores compared with scores for spontaneous tasks. J. Speech Hear. Res. 12: 875–884.

Yoss, K. A., and F. L. Darley. 1974. Developmental apraxia of speech in children with defective articulation. J. Speech Hear. Res. 17: 399–416.

Zehel, Z., R. L. Shelton, W. B. Arndt, V. Wright, and M. Elbert. 1972. Item context and /s/ phone articulation test results. J. Speech Hear. Res. 15: 852–860.

Index